OLDER SURVIVORS
OF CANCER

Older
Survivors
of Cancer

Feeling Understood by
Sharing Experiences

Alice B. Kornblith, PhD

OXFORD
UNIVERSITY PRESS

OXFORD
UNIVERSITY PRESS

Oxford University Press is a department of the University of Oxford. It furthers
the University's objective of excellence in research, scholarship, and education
by publishing worldwide. Oxford is a registered trade mark of Oxford University
Press in the UK and certain other countries.

Published in the United States of America by Oxford University Press
198 Madison Avenue, New York, NY 10016, United States of America.

CIP data is on file at the Library of Congress
ISBN 978-0-19-090203-2

9 8 7 6 5 4 3 2 1

Printed by LSC Communications, United States of America

OLDER CANCER SURVIVORS

This book is meant to be a tribute to all older cancer survivors who have withstood a battle with such a formidable opponent as cancer and came out on top. My gratitude is deep to all the participants who out of their kindness and caring for other older cancer survivors were as committed as I was to making this book happen.

JIMMIE C. HOLLAND, MD

Dr. Holland was a visionary, at the forefront of understanding the importance of quality of life issues in cancer patients' lives. She created a wide range of programs and services to enhance their lives, and trained hundreds of junior members in the cancer field to practice, expand and develop further approaches to improving their lives. Dr. Holland's reach was broad, expanding throughout the United States, and now throughout the world. That creativity, along with her total commitment and all-consuming drive throughout her professional life to improve cancer patients' lives, made her unique and irreplaceable.

ARTI HURRIA, MD

Dr. Arti Hurria began her career early on with the determination that attention must be paid to older cancer patients, in terms of both their medical care and quality of life. She considered both were essential in understanding the impact of cancer on patients' lives and developing ways to address their needs. Because of her brilliance and drive concerning older cancer patients, Dr. Hurria became an important sounding board for me as I continued to develop this book.

MY FATHER, ABRAHAM L. KORNBLITH, MD

Dedicated to my father, a General Practitioner, who was the creator of my lifelong interest in medicine.

MY MOTHER, EDNA B. KORNBLITH, AND SISTERS, PHYLLIS K. BACHELOR AND ELAINE B. JOST

Dedicated to my mother and sisters for a lifetime of their love and support.

CONTENTS

ACKNOWLEDGMENTS

Arti Hurria, MD, Vice-Provost, City of Hope; Loretta Erhunmwun-see, MD, Leslie Popplewell, MD, Sumanta Pal, MD, City of Hope; Susan Gapstur, MPH, PhD, Vice President, Epidemiology, American Cancer Society; Joanne Buzaglo, PhD, Senior Vice President of Research and Training, and Kirsten Norslien, Gilda's Club, in the Cancer Support Community; Bladder Cancer Advocacy Network; Leukemia and Lymphoma Society; Lymphoma Research Foundation; Tim Ahles, PhD, Psychiatry and Behavior Science, Memorial Sloan-Kettering Cancer Center; Erika Nalls, American Association for Cancer Research; Electra Paskett, PhD, Division of Cancer Prevention and Control, and Director of the Center for Cancer Health Equity, Ohio State University; Michelle J. Naughton, PhD, MPH, Division of Cancer Prevention and Control, Ohio State University; Christopher S. Lathan, MD, MS, MPH, Faculty Director for Cancer Care Equity, Dana-Farber Cancer Institute; Susan Goldberg; Linda Bulone, RN, Queens Hospital Cancer Center; Adriana Palmer, librarian, Graduate Center, City University of New York; Allison Piazza, librarian, New York Academy of Medicine; transcription company, iScribed.

INTRODUCTION

Why I Wrote This Book

As of 2018, there has been a major increase in not only the aging of the population, but in finding more effective treatments for cancer. As a result, in 2018, a national survey that was done in the United States found that 53.4% of cancer patients are being diagnosed with cancer when 65 years old or older (Noone et al. 2018). However, there are still fewer studies of the quality of life of *older* cancer patients and survivors than younger patients. Further, as there are many more breast cancer patients than any of the other cancers, much of the quality-of-life literature has been focused on this disease, with much less attention paid to quality-of-life issues of patients with lesser studied cancers. Consequently, the *major purpose of this book, "Older Survivors of Cancer: Feeling Understood by Sharing Experiences"*, is to reduce older cancer survivors' feeling of aloneness, of not being understood, by sharing the experiences of other older cancer survivors of their age and gender, who have the same type of cancer. Therefore, this book is likely to also be of interest to older cancer survivors' caregivers, other family members, and friends. It may increase not only their understanding of, and ability to cope with, the impact of cancer on survivors' lives, but also their understanding of how it affects their own lives as well.

I want this book to be like a conversation you might have with an older cancer survivor about how cancer affected his/her life. As a number of participants will have the same type of cancer, and will be of a similar age and gender, and will be one to five years cancer-free or in remission since their treatment ended, reading about their different experiences and ways of coping can "pack a punch." One of the participants who was interviewed may be just like you. *I hope that this book will make you feel that others understand exactly what you have gone through, making you feel less alone.* That is what this book is designed to do.

While older cancer patients and partners would be the most interested in reading *Older Survivors of Cancer,* it would also be of interest to oncologists and oncology staff members, particularly nurses, psychiatrists, psychologists, and social workers. It would likely not only increase their understanding as to how patients' quality of life has been affected by having had cancer, but also show them how to expand the ways already in place for improving patients' quality of life, and to create new ones.

Older survivors of bladder cancer, colorectal cancer, non-Hodgkin lymphoma and lung cancer were selected for this book due to the high incidence of these cancers and the interest and importance to a large number of older cancer patients and survivors. The number of people who were diagnosed with these four cancers was ranked in the top seven of all patients diagnosed with cancer in the United States in 2018. Out of a total of 1,735,350 who were diagnosed with cancer in 2018, 53% (919,735) were diagnosed at 65 years of age or older. As individuals are being diagnosed with cancer at an increasingly older age, other problems also increase, affecting their quality of life. These include: (a) an increasing number of other medical problems in addition to cancer, (b) increasing frailty, and (c) other stresses in their lives, such as getting less help and comfort from friends and relatives who have moved away, have fallen sick, or have died.

The organization of this book was inspired by the author Studs Terkel, who wrote several biographies based on survivors of major historical events, such as World War II. In *"The Good War"*, soldiers who survived the war were interviewed and their autobiographical statements were organized into the major phases of the war: during and after the war, and different aspects of the war within each phase (e.g., Germany, the Pacific). The grouping of the autobiographical statements in this way was a powerful method of conveying the experiences of soldiers for different aspects and phases of the war. This book is organized like *"The Good War"*. *Older Survivors of Cancer* includes quotes from older cancer survivors concerning their experiences of having had cancer, which are grouped by *each of the four types of cancer*, beginning with participants who are 68 years old, to the oldest participant, who is 88 years old. Under each type of cancer, their experiences are grouped into two parts, "Into and Through Treatment" and "After Treatment and Through Survivorship." Within *each* of these two parts, the quotes of different areas of quality of life are listed for each older cancer survivor. For example, "Treatment and Treatment Side Effects" and "Quality of Life During Treatment," as well as other sections, are listed under "Into and Through Treatment."

Differences in Quality of Life Between Men and Women and Between White Persons and Persons of Color (Minorities)

It was important that interviews with older cancer survivors about their quality of life include both genders for each of the four cancer diagnoses. Studies of cancer survivors have found differences in the quality of life of *men and women* cancer patients. Some studies found that men reported having a better quality of life than women. Further, in a national study, men were also found to be doing better than women due to having greater emotional, financial, and social support from family and friends (Burg et al. 2015; Adorno et al. 2017). On the other hand, women survivors of non-Hodgkin lymphoma reported that cancer had a positive impact on their lives (Sarker et al. 2017), that they had more frequently enjoyed life after treatment (Adorno et al. 2017), and that they had fewer problems concerning sexuality than did men (Cancer*Care*, 2016). Consequently, it is clear from these studies that differences in cancer patients' quality of life may be due to differences in gender, type of cancer, and/or different aspects of their lives that were affected by having cancer (such as emotional state, ability to function, and support from family and friends).

Based on the National Healthcare Quality and Disparities report of the Agency for Healthcare Research and Quality for 2017 (AHRQ 2018), the conclusion was: "Since 2003, general improvements in the quality of care have occurred. However, for *minorities*, the poor quality of care seems to persist at unacceptably higher levels compared to whites." (Green et al. 2014). In a number of studies (Green et al. 2014; Parikh-Patel et al. 2017; Fiscella and Sanders 2016), several major reasons were given to explain why non-white cancer patients had a lower quality of medical care than white cancer patients, and therefore would likely be less satisfied with their medical care: (a) racial discrimination, (b) poverty, (c) not having enough health insurance to cover the medical costs, (d) physician shortage in minority communities, which limits the access of persons of color to high quality health care, and (e) having less education. All of these situations can result in persons of color not being examined at an earlier stage and therefore, being less likely to be successfully treated (Green et al. 2014).

As there may be differences in older survivors' quality of life due to differences in the experiences of men and women, this book includes a similar number of participants in each category. A number of different ways of getting participants were tried, including consulting my colleagues who either treat minority patients or knew oncologists who treat minority patients, notification of the book in websites of large cancer organizations for each of the four cancer diagnoses in this book as well as the American Cancer Society, a national organization encompassing all types of cancer. Despite all these tactics, over a year and a half, I was not able to recruit minority participants. This might have been due to the following reasons: (a) there are significantly fewer minorities than white cancer survivors diagnosed with any of the four types of cancer included in the book; (b) minority patients are often diagnosed at a later disease stage, which reduces the likelihood of their being in remission or disease-free (one of the criteria for participation); and (c) I could not include people who do not speak English since I (who did all the interviewing) only speak English.

Value of In-Depth Telephone Interviews

Interviews with older cancer survivor participants lasted between 45 minutes and 3 hours. The length of these interviews allowed ample time for them to talk about the quality of their lives during and after treatment up to the present, how they coped with having cancer, and what advice they would give to other cancer patients and survivors about coping with this disease. Almost the entire book consists of exact quotes from the survivors' interviews, with each quote identified by a pseudonym (in order to protect their identity), their type of cancer, age, gender, and the number of years they were either cancer-free or in remission. This will let you know which participants are most like you.

What Is Needed to Keep in Mind When Reading *Older Survivors of Cancer*

The first major issue that needs to be kept in mind when reading *Older Survivors of Cancer: Feeling Understood by Sharing Experiences* is *where* older cancer survivors were found to participate. Many of the participants from organizations were found using the following ways: (a) they had participated in a large study, (b) they were in support groups, (c) they did online messaging with other cancer patients, (d) they wrote about their experiences with having cancer, which were then posted online, and (e) they responded to flyers about this book distributed to health care providers. Organizations that were used to recruit older cancer survivor participants included the Cancer Support Community, Gilda's Club, the American Cancer Society (ACS), cancer centers, and websites of specific cancer organizations for the different types of cancer, such as the Bladder Cancer Advocacy Network. Even though they may have had difficult treatments and problems in coping, some participants who joined these cancer organizations reported their cancer experiences on the their websites. Therefore, they were more likely to want to be interviewed for the book as a means for "telling their story" to other cancer patients, feeling that it could be helpful to them.

However, many older cancer survivors are very private persons, particularly about their cancer diagnoses, and don't wish to share their experiences with people they don't know. Further, resources provided by cancer organizations to cancer patients may not be available to them, for a range of reasons: (a) they are too far away or are not well enough or don't have the money to travel to an organization, support group, or lectures about cancer; and (b) don't have computers to access websites where many of the organizations include information and provide forums for users to write messages back and forth with other cancer patients.

Secondly, as many of the participants in this book report regaining some or most of their quality of life after treatment ended, it would *not* mean that most of the older cancer survivors throughout the United States would feel the same way. Even if just *one* participant in this book spoke about problems they had over the course of their cancer, it is likely that there are many older cancer survivors throughout the nation who have had the same experiences. This book would need to have a much larger number of older participants for each of the four cancer diagnoses, each gender, and all racial or ethnic groups, in order to determine exactly how many older cancer survivors in each of these groups experience a particular problem. *It is very important to keep this in mind when reading this book.*

In Sum, Older Survivor Participants' Advice to the Readers

This book may be helpful to you, when you see that older cancer survivors can understand *exactly* what you've been through. A lot of comfort can come from that. In addition, older cancer survivors provided suggestions on what was helpful to them in coping with cancer, which was the basis for their advice to others. I hope that their suggestions will be helpful to you, family members, and doctors who read this book.

Chapter 1

Older Survivors of Bladder Cancer

In 2018, bladder cancer became the sixth largest type of cancer when compared to all other cancer diagnoses in the United States. Three-quarters of bladder cancer patients were diagnosed with bladder cancer when 65 years old or older (72%). The incidence of five or more years' survival is high, as it is approximately three-quarters of bladder cancer patients (National Cancer Institute, SEER Cancer Stat Facts). The disease stage at the beginning of each older bladder cancer survivor's story has been included to identify those who were treated at an earlier disease stage (Stages I and II), as they often are, and have an easier treatment compared to those with more advanced disease (Stages III and IV).

There have been major advances in developing different types of surgery for bladder cancer patients over the past several decades, all designed to improve their quality of life. The recently established surgical treatments include removing the entire bladder (radical cystectomy) and creating (a) a new bladder (neobladder) to replace the diseased one, (b) an ileal conduit, which is an outside pouch or bag attached to the body, in which urine is collected, which has to be emptied when full, and (c) an Indiana pouch, which replaces the bladder by creating a pouch inside the body that collects the urine, and is emptied several times per day when the pouch becomes full.

Some participants in my book talked about the different surgery options that their surgeons discussed with them to consider. What was central to the participants in making this decision was, of course, which treatment would be most effective, how difficult the treatment would be, and how many and severe the side effects were, as well as the impact on continence. Incontinence was particularly noteworthy because of how it would make patients feel (diapers were an embarrassment), and restrictions it would place on their social activities, due to fears of incontinence in public. In a study involving only those who had a radical cystectomy, almost half (44%) of the patients whose bladders were entirely removed reported severe incontinence over the course of four years (Kretschmer et al. 2016). Of all the medical problems that patients endured due to treatment, Kretschmer's findings, as well as this book's participants, showed incontinence and the fear of incontinence was one of the key symptoms affecting bladder cancer survivors' quality of life.

INTO AND THROUGH TREATMENT

NANCY S.: *Non-Muscle-Invasive Bladder Cancer, Stage T1, High grade, 69 years old, female, disease-free two years*

Life One Year Before Diagnosis

I was still working as a freelance book editor: very stressful, deadline-driven job, working for myself. I'm very healthy. I've always been real active physically and had a good relationship with my husband. My kids are fine. We had a few close friends. But basically at that time, I hadn't retired, so I was working a lot. In terms of work stresses, not really. My mother was getting older and she was kind of a worry and she was showing a little dementia.

Diagnosis of Bladder Cancer

At my yearly examination with my doctor, there was some microscopic blood in the urine. I asked my doctor about it and he said, "Oh, nothing to worry about. It's probably menopause." When I came to Canada and after a while my doctor here said, "In Canada we don't let things like that go, so we're going to set you up for an appointment with the urologist and you're going to have a test." I thought it was just nothing, because I never saw any blood, I never had any symptoms, zero. The doctor ordered a cystoscopy and *(then I was diagnosed with having bladder cancer)**. I was in complete shock because I thought the cystoscopy was just a routine thing. My first thought: "Is this the way I'm going to die?" I was fortunate that there was a nurse there. She said, "You're probably not going to die of this." Possibly the worst moment of the whole deal was calling my sons and telling them I had cancer.

Treatment and Treatment Side Effects

I had to wait a month before I had my surgery and then I had to wait two weeks after that for the pathology, and I don't wait very well. That was a very, very stressful time. That was an awful time.

They put tuberculosis into your bladder. You have to hold it for two hours, and then you drink a lot of water to try and get rid of it because it's caustic. It's burning, it's pain, and you can't even hold your water for two hours. It's impossible to hold it, but you have to. For two or three days you feel like you have the flu. You're very sick, you have a temperature, and you're bleeding. When you pee, it's like peeing knives—a very sharp pain. You do that for three weeks in a row. Then you wait and get another cystoscopy. But it could have been worse than that. Chemo is worse than that. If these treatments didn't work, I would have to have an external bag on my body. I thought about that a lot and worried about that. Another person seeing a bag—that's the thing that you worry about. I didn't worry about my husband's reaction because he doesn't care.

---

* Italicized (slanted) typing is used in parentheses when quoting participants to complete their sentences, in order to make the quotes clearer.

Quality of Life During Treatment

Employment

I was working *(during treatment)*, and then I retired. Part of the reason I did was because I didn't want my time to be just working anymore. You don't have all the time in the world, and so I did retire. Also, I worked for myself so I could make that decision, and didn't need to worry about having health insurance, not keeping a job.

Relationships with Family, Friends, and Acquaintances

I sometimes think that caregivers worry more than the people with cancer. I sometimes think it's harder to be a caregiver because they feel helpless. *(My husband)* would rather have the cancer than have me have the cancer. He's frustrated because he can't really do anything. Men want to do stuff to fix things and he can't. You can't have sex pretty much during the three weeks *(while on treatment)*. Because you've got the tuberculosis (TB) bacteria *(BCG treatment for bladder cancer is a germ related to tuberculosis)*, I think that someone could get TB. You don't want to pass it to another person. After a couple of days you can resume *(having sex)*.

When people hear the word *(cancer)*, they just shut down and they don't listen past that. I found it difficult to talk about it because people just look at you with such long, drawn faces and then you're treated differently. It's kind of like they don't want to get too close to you because you could be contagious. Some people think that you bring it on yourself, like lung cancer. Some people think it's a heroic thing *(to fight cancer)* and that you're a trooper. I have to say the thing I hate the most is when people talk about a battle. So, they say, "You're fighting cancer. You're a warrior." What that means to me is that if you don't live, then there is something you did, which is bullshit, because it's cancer. Cancer got you. It wasn't because you didn't fight hard enough. I don't like the militaristic part of that.

Social Life

When I first got cancer and the whole thing was going on, there was a lot going on at the beginning. I was kind of bored of social groups. I quit some things because I just wanted to only do things that were really important to me.

Coping with Having Cancer

I sort of got objective about it and looked at it as a project that I was going to learn as much as I could. That gives you a little distance between you and the disease. The more I learned, the more powerful I felt. As I was a librarian and liked research, I just did as much research as I possibly could and taught myself the jargon, reading medical journal articles. The one thing I wanted was to be able to talk to Dr. B and my other doctors as a person who halfway understood what they were talking about. When you have cancer, it's like all the controls are gone. You're just like this pawn in this cancer machine. This is what's going to happen, you're going to wait, you're going to always wait and it's awful. The little bit of control I had was having as much knowledge as I could get as a layperson, so that I could ask the right questions. As soon as I started doing that, I joined the Bladder Cancer Advocacy Network (BCAN) and some other forums, and started talking to other people. That really made a huge difference, because they started telling me about their experience and their story.

Coping Needs That Went Unmet

I needed something like my friends with breast cancer have, which is a huge organization of people and support.

Satisfaction with Medical Care During Treatment

I have to applaud the Canadian health care system because I think it saved my life. If I had waited longer, and I think even if I had just waited a little bit longer, I would have had muscle invasive bladder cancer, which is very serious. But when you have non-muscle-invasive, it means it's still sitting on the bladder wall and it's not on its way to invading any other parts of your body. In that way it's a "good cancer."

I had the best doctor in the whole world. I didn't have to worry. I didn't have to second guess what he was doing. *(MD, RN, Health Care Team)* were surely caring, very compassionate. They let you be emotional. I was free to be as neurotic as I wanted to be. But I had to go and be my own advocate. My urologist is always too busy—didn't have the time. I had to go and make time to find out, to get answers to my questions. What I did for example is that there is a nurse that works with my doctor and the urology team. I've gotten to know her and I did this on purpose. She gave me her own private number. She's been there a million years. She probably knows as much as the docs. I've called her and I've talked to her and she takes time with me. But that's something I had to do. It's not given to you. If you're shy, or if you're one of those kind of people that doesn't want to know a lot, you're not going to get it.

MILLY H.: *Bladder Cancer, Stage II, 70 years old; female, disease-free four years*

Life One Year Before Diagnosis

Life was great. I was in about my fifth year of retirement. I had found hobbies to do that I'd never get time to do in the past. I learned how to work with wood and I was making bowls and vases and Christmas ornaments, going to craft shows, just having a wonderful time with that. Then I picked up quilting which was something I had done as a youngster with my mother but let it slide. I was fishing, I was hunting, I was hiking. I have always been very active. I love to be outside a whole lot, more than I love to be inside. I spend a lot of hours gardening in the summer and then putting up the vegetables, making soup for the winter. I was having a great time. My husband and I were doing well even though he's always had a lot of problems with depression and anxiety but we were coping with each other being so different. I was always looking at the bright side, he was always looking at the not-so-bright side, but we were doing well.

(In the year before my diagnosis) I broke my pelvis. That affected me mentally probably more than anything else because it was very depressing—not to be able to hike, not to be able to get up stairs to my sewing machine, not to be able to turn around. But again I had a friend who said, "Milly, let's join the Y *(YMCA)*. I know you can't do anything else, but you can swim." So we went and joined the Y. Exercise is my best defense against stress, anxiety, and depression. And so, if you can't walk, swim.

Diagnosis of Bladder Cancer

I was probably the most frightened the day my doctor gave me the official diagnosis after the biopsy results from the TURBT *(transurethral resection of the bladder tumor)*. It was probably the most frightened I ever felt. My husband, now my ex-husband, was not very good with words but he just held me and said, "We'll get through this," which was a big help. Fortunately, I hooked up early on with some people who shared very good information with me. I was fairly well convinced by the time that I got my diagnosis, that it wasn't a death sentence. It did not have to be a death sentence. I kept it from my children until I got that final diagnosis even though they were aware that I was concerned about the blood in my urine.

Treatment and Treatment Side Effects

I started four months of chemo, Cisplatin and Gemzar. I had really bad reactions to the first chemotherapy. My blood counts were so terribly low. My immune system was terribly weak. I had to wear a mask and wash my hands constantly. They reduced the dose of Cisplatin and Gemzar by 13% and along with Neulasta *(increases immunity to germs)* I was able to get through chemo.

Quality of Life During Treatment

Relationships with Family, Friends, and Acquaintances

My family was amazing. I have three sons and one of those sons was with me for the entire four months of chemo, namely because they knew that my husband was not very good at doing things for me. He was very supportive but he was kind of a helpless kid. My sons knew he couldn't cook for me, so they were there. They were there for the entire time and that is probably the thing that helped me get through chemo, more than anything else. They helped me keep my garden up. I thought I just wouldn't be able to do this, because it was the main gardening season, May through September. But the thing that helped me the most was my sister and her constant reminder that people all over the world were praying for me. She had put out the word to every person she knew, to every mission she supported, until there were people all over the world praying for me. On days when it was warm enough to go outside, my sister put blankets around me and she'd take me outside to sit in the sunshine because I'm a sunshine person. Just her recognizing what I needed to keep a positive outlook of life is one of the biggest things that pulled me through, and of course my children calling constantly.

Sexual Life

(My husband and I) didn't have sex, but we had not been having sex for a couple of years before all this started because he had problems in that area. So he chose to stop having sex about two years before any of this ever came up. So I frankly don't think my bladder cancer and any of the health problems after that had any effect on our sex life, because we already had no sex life.

Religion

I have grappled with my faith, all of my life. I've gone beyond thinking, "Well I'm an agnostic; I don't really believe." But all the things that happened in that year convinced me that God was looking out for me.

Satisfaction with Medical Care During Treatment

I had excellent doctors throughout, dealing with my cancer. When my urologist told me it would be six weeks before I could have my TURBT done, I told him I could not wait that long. I told him the stress would kill me and patience was never my strong suit. He found a way to do it two weeks later. He and his PA *(Physician Assistant)* were amazing. They gave me cell phone numbers and email addresses so I could get in touch with them with any questions. My doctor and the staff at *(the medical center)* took such good care of me and still do take care of me. I think all the people who treated me made sure I had everything I needed to get me back to my active lifestyle. There are such amazing people in the hospital, from the nurses all the way down to the custodians. They were constantly saying and doing things to encourage me to get better. They even threw me a birthday party because I was in the hospital for my birthday. The whole staff came in and sang "Happy Birthday" to me on my birthday. From the top person on 11 West to the custodian, they all took care of me.

JOE C.: *Bladder Cancer, Stage IV, 72 years old, male, disease-free two years*

Life One Year Before Diagnosis

I'm happily married with my wife, and our son and his wife were living in town. We just had a brand new grandbaby. We were in high heaven. I've been pretty much healthy all of my life. My wife and I have always been involved in an active life. We're just active, fit people and didn't really worry much about our health. My wife and I also had traveled widely. We were getting older. I was also burned out of energy for having been in so many places.

Diagnosis of Bladder Cancer

I had blood in my urine. *(After the cystoscopy, the doctor)* was absolutely certain at that point that it was a cancer in my bladder. I was just kind of stunned. I've been so healthy all my life. I was not really anticipating it would be bad, bad news.

Treatment and Treatment Side Effects

The idea of having the external pouch *(where urine flows to an external pouch through an opening in the wall of the abdomen)* was something I just didn't want to do. It just seems so cumbersome. I've never liked anything sticking to my skin. I've never had any experience with adhesives that I'm supposed to stick to myself, and the idea of having it in the same place on my body for the rest of my life was just a dreadful idea to me.

Before the surgery, I had all these other TURBTs *(transurethral resection of the bladder tumor)* and procedures. They would lay me low for a short period of time and then I'd be right back to normal functioning. When I got to the actual major surgery to the neobladder *(bladder was removed, and a new bladder was created from the small intestine)*, I was just totally incapacitated for a while. It was a real ordeal physically and logistically for the first three weeks. I came home after being released from the hospital but then I needed to go back for three more weekly visits after that. The first three weeks after I came home I was still using a catheter bag and giving myself injections. Every six hours, 24/7, I was supposed to flush the neobladder through the catheter and do a saline flush to clear out the mucus *(slimy substance which moistens and protects surfaces, such as the bladder)*, and debris. There's no way I could have done that by myself. I was so wiped out physically. Wonderful friends volunteered to drive us down and back to the hospital each time we had to go because my wife didn't feel good driving with just her and me in the car. She thought I might need attending to at any moment. That whole process of going to the hospital and doing the TURBT and then another one and coming home with the catheter bag and trying to drag everything around the house, and function like a human being during that recovery process, was pretty taxing. It was a first for me, in terms of really being stuck with something in my life that was very, very difficult medically to just shake off.

It took a long time for me to get my regular digestive function back. The antibiotics and the anesthetics really did a job on my digestive tract. That was a big problem. There was quite a bit of minor leakage just from body movements if I sneezed or coughed or if I had to bend suddenly. We bought some basic pull-on incontinence underpants. You just wear them under regular pants. I think it was probably eight weeks after the surgery that I started to have reasonable control *(over leakage of urine)*. I was just wearing adult diapers all the time which is a horrible thing to do. I wore those for a time and then transitioned to just having a pad. It took about three or four months of that before I had enough confidence to not wear the pad all the time.

Non-Cancer Medical Problems

I had osteopenia before I started chemo and all of the steroids that they gave me made it progress immediately to osteoporosis *(brittle and fragile bones)*. It was so bad that I was getting little fractures in my pubic bone that made it difficult to walk. So my oncologist has me taking a Prolia shot every six months and my bone density has improved. But I think that's going to be something I always struggle with. But that's why I'm doing so much hiking and walking and weightlifting at the gym to try to stave off *(osteoporosis)* as much as I can. But I understand there will be a time in my life where I probably won't be able to walk and I won't be able to lift those weights. And so the osteoporosis is going to progress and get worse.

Quality of Life During Treatment

Emotional State

Prior to surgery I tried to be as cool as I could be and do what was necessary. I was still really hopeful that this will be a one-shot deal, like they'd take the tumor out and that would be the end of it. My whole attitude through this process was that I tried to avoid dreading things, to be as informed as I could. The biggest problem I had with pain was the TURBT. Just having the catheter was really uncomfortable, pulling it around. More emotionally painful I think because I felt like I was a big burden to everybody around me.

If I allowed myself to dread things after surgery, *(the dreading would be)* worse than the reality. So I tried to keep that in mind. You're in such embarrassing, bizarre circumstances so often. You just kind of get over that. Because I had essentially almost a year's worth of dealing with TURBTs, going in and out of the hospital before the big surgery, I became accustomed to that pretty quickly. I could view it humorously and there was a certain degree of detachment. I didn't have a great deal of problems adjusting, but that whole ominous notion that you're going to be incontinent for the rest of your life and having to deal with draining yourself all the time with emptying the bags, that was tough. In the long run, that was the difficult fear that I had.

Relationships with Family, Friends, and Acquaintances

(On hearing the urologist's recommendation that I have the radical cystectomy), my poor wife was like "Our lives are over." That was a really despairing moment for both of us. I was just numb through the whole procedure of checking into the hospital and the signing all the papers, and showing up early in the morning and doing the whole thing. My wife was very, very, very distraught. She was anticipating the end of life as we knew it. She wasn't sure she could deal with the burden of what was going to be expected of her as the caretaker in the immediate aftermath. She soldiered through and I think she suffered emotionally more than I did. *(When I was discharged from the hospital after the surgery)* we started the three-week routine of having to flush *(the bladder)* every six hours, which is a real nasty thing you have to face. To do it yourself would just have been an overwhelming task, in terms of how exhausted and easily fatigued I was. Her help was essential. *(My son)* was totally helpful. He and his family were

really concerned. He was positive all the way throughout, and that was good.

Friends were terrific. I just told them "here's the situation" and shared with them whatever they wanted to know. I'm just going to be open and tell people what's going on and hope for the best. I think that served me well. I was really fortunate to have two very, very good friends who served as role models for me. They're physically disabled now, but they had to deal with pain and overcoming physical issues that were way beyond any of the physical challenges I've been dealt with. They still have done what they wanted to do. That was an inspiration to me and I decided that was the way I needed to go. When a good friend found out that I was having surgery, she said, "I've got the Poor Clare Nuns *(nunnery in Santa Barbara)* praying for you. They're really good." It was a good thing that they were doing that. *(Having)* direct face-to-face experience with two radical cystectomy veterans *(one with a neobladder, the other with an external pouch)* was a crucial factor in my decision-making process and mental preparation *(for the upcoming surgery).*

Satisfaction with Medical Care During Treatment

The doctor was just adamant that there's no way you should do the *(surgery)* here *(smaller hospital)*, because you should go to the *(medical center)* or any of the other National Cancer Institute (NCI) hospitals where they do these surgeries several times a week. They have the facilities and the expertise to do it.

(At the medical center) I had a really good relationship with my urologist. She was very sharp and very blunt. I like that she didn't have any hesitation to tell people what she thought or what she thought should be done. We trusted her a great deal and we felt like she was always going to be straightforward with us. She sat down with us and got a piece of paper out and just drew a flow chart saying "Look, you've got bladder cancer. We're going to do this TURBT. If the results go this way, then we'll do this next. If the result goes the

other way, then we'll do this next." I'll then know both sides of that possibility. That took a lot of mystery out of what would probably happen. The surgeons were very good about communicating with my wife about what was going on with the surgery. About every 45 minutes or hour, they would call her and say, "Everything's going OK so far" and just reassure her that everything was on track. She felt very good about the level of communication that was happening.

I do think the doctors were personable and they cared about my welfare. I think they did everything extraordinarily well. I didn't feel as if I was ever depersonalized by them. My doctors were exceptionally upbeat and informative at all stages. I didn't expect them to go beyond that in assuaging my anxiety. Rather, I relied on friends and family. Because I was always aware of other options and next steps during the lead up to the radical cystectomy surgery, and because the outcome has been very positive, I never faced real depression.

MIKE S.: *Bladder Cancer, Stage T1, 73 years old, male, disease-free one year*

Life One Year Before Diagnosis

At this time last year, I was eating celery and sipping rice. This time now, I'm drinking Scotch, having pasta, enjoying my family, having a ball. I've been very fortunate because, health-wise, I've never had a problem and the only thing I really had to take was a cholesterol pill.

Diagnosis of Bladder Cancer

Between 70 and 71 years old, I noticed that I was going to the bathroom more and more and it was getting a little uncomfortable. Then I went to see the doctor in the hospital and he felt that I had an overactive bladder, so he did a minor surgery. Then what happened was it kept being a problem and then, all of a sudden, one morning, I got up and I urinated all blood. The next morning, the same thing happened. *(My oncologist)* took the x-rays and did all the CAT scans and he felt that there were tumors of cancer in my bladder. He didn't know the extent, but then when he went in, he told me my whole bladder was infested with cancer. I was shocked that I had bladder cancer.

Treatment and Treatment Side Effects

Then last December 13 was a four-and-a-half hour neobladder surgery where they removed my bladder *(and created a new bladder from the small intestine)*. I had stitches right down the middle of my stomach and I had the catheter. There was no pain at all. It was just more discomfort with the stitches down the middle of my stomach and with the catheter. Just the thought of taking a shower, that I took for granted, was a struggle. It was a struggle to turn in bed because in sleeping with the catheter I had to sleep on my back. I felt sorry for myself for about 12 hours and that was it, because I was determined to keep going and I am. Once the catheter was taken out, there was no problem. That was such a relief. That was the most discomfort.

Then my wife would irrigate it every four hours and that lasted for about six weeks. Once the stitches healed and the catheter was removed, then it was just a matter of doing what I had to do: walking, climbing stairs, watching what I was eating, and just behaving. Each time I went back to *(the doctor)* every three months, he kept saying there was progress. After a year, he said that I was cancer-free. I could resume my 10-pound weights, and he let me do sit-ups. Now, after a year, I feel like a whole new person.

(Because of incontinence) we had these little portable diapers. If I was going to a function, I would wear them for security. I'd rather be safe than sorry if I was going to take the train down to a movie or a Broadway play or some type of function. Now that's completely eliminated.

Maybe the most difficult experience was at the beginning *(of treatment)* because I couldn't do things, like taking out the garbage and not being able to empty the dishwasher. Because of the stitches there, I couldn't bend and lift anything. Then what happened was the garbage guys saw that my wife was taking the garbage out, so they said, "Forget about it, just leave it in the driveway," and they picked it up. There was all this goodness all around.

Quality of Life During Treatment

Emotional State

At first there were a couple of tears and I felt sorry for myself. Then I said to myself, "Hold on now. Let's be a big boy here." Because I was 72 years old at the time and my granddaughter was four, I said, "You know what? That's going to be my motivation. I want to see her grow up, I want to be part of her life."

Relationships with Family, Friends, and Acquaintances

My wife's a strong person. She just knew what she had to do, and the nurse taught her how to irrigate me. It was like having a real nurse with my wife. I have to go now for treatment for an erection *(prostate was removed at the time of the bladder surgery)*. We had to wait a year and now I have an appointment in January to see whether some type of needle or a pill or whatever will enable me to resume my sexual life. *(This didn't affect my relationship with my wife)* because we're in this together. We've been married 48 years. I've got two great daughters, everyone has been so good to me. I love them dearly—great kids. One is 47 and one is 46 years old. When I got sick, it was like they became seven years old and six years old again, they were so good. The younger one would come in the morning, the older one would come in the afternoon.

I had great support from everybody: the guys I'd worked with, the guys I taught with, my real estate, my neighbors. It was fantastic. Just the phone calls, the cookies, the flowers, the constant concern for me and love for me and what they could do at any time. People couldn't do enough for us. When people found out *(that I had bladder cancer)*, they would call and say, "What can I do?" It was like a tidal wave.

Satisfaction with Medical Care During Treatment

(The cancer center) was very, very good. The other thing is that they have a 24-hour service, so anytime there was a question that my wife had, there was a doctor on duty that would answer the question. That was it. Then the visiting nurses, they came like twice a week when I was home, and they were very positive and very good.

The anxiety level was there, but my doctor was very reassuring, gave us all his plans for surgery. He said the thing you've got to do now is you got to keep moving because you don't want the blood clots or anything else to form. I get in the room, an hour later, I was walking around the halls and doing what he said. I got out of the hospital in two and a half days and then I was able to do everything he's wanted me to do. I feel like a million dollars because every time I see my little granddaughter, that smile keeps going. That's incentive. Now this Christmas with her, at five years old, was a thing of beauty, it was so much fun.

With my stitches, the bottom stitch—talking about the help you would get—the bottom stitch kept leaking. So what happened was my wife called down to *(the cancer center)* and they told me to pick up this Medihoney *(honey product used for the management of acute and chronic wounds and burns)*. It's like a little cream and once she rubbed that on, that stopped the leaking. So there was always help. Any question we had, they always had the answers.

SHARRON O.: *Bladder Cancer, Stage IV, 76 years old, female, disease-free one year*

Life One Year before Diagnosis

I was very busy. I was working very long hours. Very much involved in my community, and, to some extent with my children. My children are all grown and most of my grandchildren have grown too, so I don't have a lot of day-to-day contact with them. My great-grandsons live in another county, so I don't necessarily have day-to-day contact with them either. But I did have frequent contact either by telephone or in-person. It was a very busy, full life. Many years ago, I had been in a domestic violence situation and one of the discs in my back was out of place. A couple of years after that, there was a very much increased issue of frequent urination that was actually tied to that disc being out of place.

Diagnosis of Bladder Cancer

I was walking across the parking lot and tripped over the cement curb, and I fell landing on my elbow, which shattered my elbow and shoulder. I was in surgery, getting my elbow put back together. In the battery of tests they ran before the surgery, the GP *(General Practitioner)* called me the day before surgery and said, "there's blood in your urine and we need to determine where it's coming from." *(After an ultrasound and biopsy, the doctor)* sat me down and said he could say for sure that there was cancer in my bladder, and he was quite certain that it was Stage IV cancer, and that it would have gone into the muscle and probably some of the lymph nodes surrounding it.

The biopsy was on September 26 and my actual major surgery for cancer was on October 21. I was kind of walking in a fog by this time since things were just moving very quickly. My whole focus was on being able to listen to what they were saying, taking notes about what I needed to do, what my choices were, so that I could go back and look at it again to make sure I had understood it correctly. It was like a roller coaster. I went for the ultrasound and then I was into another whole system where I ended up with the biopsy, which put me in another whole system at *(the medical center)*. It was literally 60 days from the first time I saw Dr. R, the gynecologist, until I was in surgery for 12 hours to have the surgery for cancer.

I think it was beneficial for me to not have everyone in the family floating around asking questions and telling you what they thought. I do have this friend of mine with me, but basically her role as she saw it was to make sure I got where I needed to be, to take copious notes on what the doctors were saying so that if I forgot something, I could go back and check her notes. But it wasn't her place to tell me what to do; that was my decision.

Treatment and Treatment Side Effects

They removed the bladder, uterus, ovaries, cervix, and I believe something like 32 lymph nodes. I have a stoma and external bag. I had one main incision down the center that's probably four inches long and a couple of the staples had come out of that and the fluid was leaking out through that incision. What they ended up doing was taking essentially a sanitary napkin, cutting it in half and placing it over the incision to absorb the fluid as it came out. I would change that every couple of hours because it would fill up. This went on for six or eight weeks. My focus was on this stuff coming out of my stomach. *(It seemed that the cause was the in-home health care worker)* who was in a little bit of a hurry and pulled the sanitary napkin off. There was an open lesion and it hadn't been treated. While the flow through the incision was diminishing, it still meant I couldn't really go anywhere because I leaked. There was no way to stop the leaking other than what you could absorb with this pad. I ended up going back to *(the medical center)* and it became a once-a-week thing. I would go in, they would take off the bag, look at the incision and cauterize the incision—it hurt a lot. It did eventually heal. It took a very, very long time.

Quality of Life During Treatment

Emotional State

One of my very best experiences came from a friend of mine who had a colostomy bag *(used to collect BMs for colorectal cancer patients who had part of their colon removed)* many years ago. We got together after my surgery and she was talking about the first time that you feel motion on your skin, and you don't know what it is, and it feels like there's a bug crawling on you because you're still kind of a little groggy from the medicine. When I felt the warm liquid moving along inside this bag, it felt very strange. The first time that you realize what it is, it really is kind of scary. Now, I just kind of laugh at it.

Relationships with Family, Friends, and Acquaintances

Most of my kids are pretty stable about this: "We'll get through this and just take it day by day." I did not want all of them at the hospital. I have four kids plus any number of others who would like to have been there. It would be like anywhere from six to ten people sitting around in the waiting room for 14 hours. It just did not make sense to me at all. They designated my oldest son to be there and he was there when I went into surgery in the morning, as was the woman who has my power-of-attorney. They were there when I came out.

(My daughter) was fighting with every bit of her being to not panic about *(my)* going to be dead in six months. That was her experience *(when she was helping to take care of her father/my ex-husband)*. She tried really, really hard and she stayed away from me unless she was OK and could pull it off. I think that's true of literally everyone in your world. They all have an experience, and that's how they relate to you. They ask questions that are intrusive, annoying, scary. They don't mean to be a problem. They mean to be helpful. But it's just

more stress to be dealing with a body that's already stressed because it's been through so much. I have another daughter who I don't talk to a lot and avoided at that point in time, but I was furious because she had told her family that this was very serious, it was a major operation, and I might not live through the operation. I was like, "OK, we're not going to talk to you for six months. I don't need this."

A friend of mine called me two or three days after the surgery and said, "My daughter tells me that I'm supposed to get on a plane and go take care of you." *(My friend)* had been here a few weeks *(ago)* at the time of the initial fall. She then came back right after the surgery for cancer and she stayed here for probably three or four weeks. She's the one who looked and said, "This is stupid. You're oozing stuff. We're taking you to the hospital." I could not have done it by myself simply because even if I had strength, there was this stuff oozing and it was coming out so fast.

Coping with Having Cancer

I think *(the pain)* was there. I just tend to avoid pain. I don't have time for it, because pain is going to get me down and I don't want to be down. *(My dog)* would lie at my feet and kind of look at me like, "You have a problem. Why? I'm not going anywhere. I'm staying here with you." But he was really neat because if nobody else was around, I could sit and talk to him, and he would look at me like he understood what I was saying.

Satisfaction with Medical Care During Treatment

(The medical center) is just an incredibly wonderful facility. The doctors are really, really good at what they do and you know that when you talk to them. They're very explicit. They can answer every question you have. If they don't know the answer, they will tell you they don't know, which is kind of comforting in a way. The care in the hospital was absolutely exemplary, and the food was anything that you wanted. There was a pullback bed if someone wanted to stay in the

room with me. There were three nurses that are basically room care nurses, but they do a whole lot of other stuff too. They're your security blanket from surgery on. They came, in turns, during the day, to make sure everything was OK. There was a physical therapist who came in to find out if I was going to need anything. If that were the case, they would start that immediately. There was a case manager who was going to be in charge of getting all my supplies put together. They even had a woman come in who helped me take a shower and wash my hair two days after surgery. I felt fortunate to have the very best services provided to me. *(The medical center)* has personnel to cover just about every need and question, and they are all readily available.

My new best friends at *(the medical center)* were my three wound care nurses, because I saw them once a week and they dealt with this all the time. I have not seen them since my incision healed. Every once in a while when I'm going back for my follow-up appointments with either the surgeon or the oncologist, I run into one of them and it's like an old home week, with hugs and kisses.

SCOTT: *Bladder Cancer, Early Stage, 79 years old, male, disease-free one year*

Life One Year Before Diagnosis

I was working full-time and full-time in our business was never 9:00 to 5:00. It was more like 8:00 to 7:00 or something like that. I was the president of the Homeowners Association where I live. I am an Eagle Scout and I've been active for years with the Boy Scouts of America. I had a very full life. Emotionally I was feeling pretty good.

Diagnosis of Bladder Cancer

I have some kidney problems as a result of an allergic reaction to a medication. I do have some cardiac issues, bradycardia *(low heartbeat)* and kidney disease, but not anything that would put me on my back. Other than that, I was physically fine except for some urinary issues. I was getting up three or four times a night to urinate. That was the only thing that was a deterrent in my life. I talked to my primary care doctor who recommended that I see a local urologist.

We made an appointment for *(the local urologist)* to do a cystoscopy in his office. When he was finished he said, "I wish I could say happy birthday *(my birthday was that day)*, but unfortunately you have a bladder full of cancer." He felt certain that at that point the cancer was fully contained and in my bladder. He wanted me to try this therapy with something called BCG (Bacillus Calmette-Guerin). He did try to be very reassuring about the fact that he felt that this was at a very early stage. He didn't feel that it was life threatening at this point. "We can treat the bladder cancer and you wouldn't have any other problems, but you can't waste any time." Then *(my girlfriend)* explained a lot of things to me about the fact that the cancer is self-contained, and as long as the cancer stays in the bladder I wasn't going to have to worry about getting lung cancer or kidney cancer or liver cancer. Having a person like that in your life is a very good thing.

When you hear that you have cancer, the first thing that pops in your head is death. *(I thought about my father)* who died from cancer. I thought about people that I knew that had had some type of cancer and are dead now. Initially, you hear "cancer," and think of it as a death sentence. I called *(my friend)* who was very reassuring: "Don't get in the car and drive and think you're a dead man." That was the very first day. I didn't say anything to anybody at that point. But I did have a little bit of trouble digesting it.

(Given that I had bradycardia and kidney disease), all my medical friends told me that I had to go to a university hospital, so that if something did happen, they would have the facilities to get me a cardiologist, get me this, get me that, and they would be there in a heartbeat.

Treatment and Treatment Side Effects

(After the BCG treatment was completed and several cystoscopies had been done, the urologist) said, "The cancer is not gone and you're going to need surgery." The suggestion was that they remove the bladder because they felt 99% certain that the cancer was still contained in my bladder. *(The type of surgery chosen out of three options)* was to have an external bag. *(The urologist said)* "When we remove the bladder, we fix everything up inside so that you will have a small, external bag, essentially a new penis. It's going to come out of your tummy. You wear a band and you just wear the urostomy bag for the rest of your life. You change it every day or so." I felt a little bit apprehensive with having to deal with the urostomy bag. And when I say apprehensive, I mean having to change it myself, instead of having help in a hospital or help with the visiting nurses who were initially taking care of the wound at my home.

Quality of Life During Treatment

Emotional State

I was thinking positive, that the treatment (BCG) was going to work and because the doctors said "we did find it early." I was disappointed that BCG didn't work. Surgery itself *(which was the next treatment)* didn't scare me. What scared me is the anesthesia part, because I always had this deep seated feeling that I'm going to go to sleep and never wake up. Of course, I was anxious the first ten days before we got the pathology results. *(The pathology report showed that)* the cancer was completely gone.

Relationships with Family, Friends, and Acquaintances

My girlfriend was 100% supportive. She was part of all these discussions because she is a nurse. She deals with cancer every day.

I wanted her opinion and I wanted her to be part of the decision process. *(When I was in the hospital)* Linda wasn't there every day, but she was there a lot. My son lives about 10 minutes away from me. Between him and his wife and my oldest grandson, they came to say hello. My grandson came to see me pretty much every day. *(My children)* have their own lives, but if Linda couldn't handle something, they did. I do have a lot of friends who popped in and out. There is nobody in my life who told me that "because you have cancer, I don't want to bother with you anymore." Everybody has been totally supportive: my friends, my brothers, the rest of my family, everybody.

Sexual Life

Probably for five years before all this *(bladder cancer)* happened, my sex life was pretty limited in terms of intercourse. I related it to the fact that I had diabetes, high blood pressure, and was on medication. *(Not being able to have sex)* was very important. It's something that I have just learned to live with, which essentially I did.

Employment

It kind of pissed me off because you work with these people. It's not like I worked in an office with 150 people. We were a group of nine people and of the nine, six of them *(I've known)* for the whole seven years. *(After the surgery, my boss said)*, "Take another week and don't rush yourself and come in that Monday after." On Saturday morning, he called me, and told me that the company had essentially eliminated my position and that I was not to come in on Monday and I would get a severance package details by FedEx on Tuesday. This is the guy that I worked under directly for seven years. We socialized together. We used to go out to dinner. Linda and I would meet him and his wife. We had dinner when we worked at the other company. It was more of a relationship than just employee-boss. He *(now)* tells me, "Essentially, you're done."

Religion

Other than God got me through this, religion played no role as far as I was concerned.

Other Medical Problems

(First), a pacemaker was put in because of the bradycardia and *(the doctors)* cauterized areas that can cause AFib *(irregular heartbeat that can lead to heart failure and a stroke)*. I did feel better—more bounce to the ounce. *(Second)*, my kidney doctor told me that I have to really work at keeping my potassium down, so I don't eat potatoes, tomatoes, and bananas. I'm a meat-and-potatoes guy. But, by and large, I'm very good *(in following this diet)*.

Coping with Having Cancer

My girlfriend *(who helped me cope)* is far and away Number 1. When I was hospitalized after this surgery, my brother and his wife stayed with me for two days, which was great. And, of course, my son, daughter, and two grandkids are down here. My older grandson was totally interested in everything that was going on. My dog is very important. He's my buddy. I take him everywhere.

Satisfaction with Medical Care During Treatment

(In discussing the surgery with another surgeon and doctor, they felt that) given my underlying cardiac and kidney issues, they strongly suggested that I not even think about having a surgery like this in essentially a local community hospital. I needed to be in a university hospital setting where if they needed a cardiologist, they can have one at the drop of a hat. If they needed a nephrologist, they could have one at the drop of a hat, and so on.

When the *(medical center)* initially admitted me, I was on a different floor and they were not very good with IVs. When I finally got to the urology floor, those people knew what they were doing with everything. They were a great bunch. Dr. G *(urology surgeon at a university hospital)* was wonderful. The nephrology *(kidney)* team, the cardiac *(heart)* team, the urology *(bladder)* team were all terrific. The guy I saw more than anybody else was a resident on Dr. G's team. He was available anytime, knowledgeable. Being a patient at *(the medical center)*, I would recommend it to anybody. The nurses there are terrific. If you hit your buzzer, you don't sit and wait 20 minutes before somebody comes in. Somebody will come in within two or three minutes. It may be an aide, a tech or a nurse. Somebody responds.

PAULINE N.: *Bladder Cancer, Stage IV, 81 years old, female, disease-free one year*

Life One Year Before Diagnosis

I own a nursing home and was the director of nurses. Life was pretty good. However, even like a year ago, I knew there was something wrong physically. I felt like I was more tired and I couldn't do as much as I *(had done before)*. I'm a nurse and I know about cancer. I know what happens, but I bet people just really basically do not want to know until it just hits you right straight in the face. I smoked most of my life and I knew that I could get cancer of the bladder, but I just figured I would never get it. I just lived in denial. *(A medical problem)* I had was back pain, which was diagnosed as spinal stenosis. A noninvasive procedure was done, but it did not help me. I had pain constantly. I couldn't walk very far. My balance was good, but it was just painful to stand for a long time. I had injections in my spine and that helped for about three to four months. Then the pain would gradually come back. I always liked to look nice and dress nice. I never let myself go. Nobody really basically knew how I felt. Even though I couldn't walk far, my life was not limited. I had lots of friends. Dealing with the people in the nursing home was the greatest help in the world because you give so much of yourself over there, and you'll forget about yourself.

Diagnosis of Bladder Cancer

About a year before I was diagnosed, I was really compromised physically already. I felt like I couldn't do as much as I did before. I was tired all the time. I totally did not face it. Cancer went through my head a little bit, but it was put out of my consciousness real fast. Then, toward the end of the year, I started having some blood clots come up. I did have some tests done, but I didn't go to the right people. They did not know. I would get a couple of clots coming out and I said, "This is not normal. Something is going on in here." Then I had to go to the emergency room and the diagnosis was made. I was devastated.

Treatment and Treatment Side Effects

The next thing that had to be done was to take the tumor out. With this type of thing, there's no fear, it's just happening. If you don't make it, then you don't make it. I myself never thought there was no hope. Another doctor said that I'm going to have to have the entire bladder taken out and my uterus removed. I felt, why in the world would they want to take the whole bladder out? That would mean I would get an external pouch (*a rerouting of urine to an external pouch through an opening in the wall of the stomach [stoma]*). I tried everything to not have it done. Having an external pouch was not new to me. I've worked on patients in my nursing home who have had external pouches. I didn't think I would ever get used to it. As the tumor was growing on one of the urethras, I had chemotherapy. The only big problem I had was a lot of cramping in my colon. It was quite painful. It lasted maybe less than a week.

Quality of Life During Treatment

Emotional State

I thought, after surgery, I'm going to get over this and move on. I was not really thinking what the future would hold. It was like a step by step. If I survive, it would be great. I was mad, not depressed.

Relationship with Family, Friends, and Acquaintances

My children felt that they weren't going to lose me because I'm the only thing that they have. Even if they're older, with some of them who are in their 50s, they were very attached to me. They were very sad.

Coping with Having Cancer

I didn't need (*anything to help me cope with having cancer that I didn't get*). I didn't ask for any of it (*e.g., support groups*). If I had asked, I'm sure they would have provided that, because they just basically have almost everything. At least they would have directed me where to go.

Satisfaction with Medical Care During Treatment

I went to the best (*medical center*) that I knew. I would not deal with any other doctor or with any other people except (*the medical center*) because I have so much faith in them. The nurses were so kind and understanding. They always had a smile for you. I never saw a cross employee. You're not afraid to ask them a question. If you have an accident, something happens, you're not afraid to call a nurse. They are the nicest people, from the people directing the place, or the nurse that takes your blood pressure, or the man that is going to say. "I will help you find the room. Can I push your wheelchair?"

(*After the surgery, my oncologist*) said that I should go on hospice, that there was absolutely nothing else that they can do for me. He said that I had three months to live and that the maximum maybe six. I said to him, "Really? You filleted me like a fish. You took everything out inside of me and now you're telling me there's nothing else you can do? You don't do this kind of surgery to a person and then you tell them to go on hospice. I don't believe you. You figure out what you're going to do for me." Yes, there was a kindness and caring *(in this oncologist)*. He didn't say that because he was not caring. He said that because that's what he believed. I totally admire the doctor. He works very hard. He does research. He tries to help the human race to see if we can fight this disease somehow.

TERRY TUPPER: *Bladder Cancer, Stage I, Grade 4, 85 years old, female, disease-free one year*

Life One Year Before Diagnosis

I had no medical problems. I am very fit. I walk about 50 miles a week and I exercise every day. Eighteen months prior to being diagnosed with bladder cancer I was selling my property that my husband and I had bought when we moved out here to Wisconsin. That meant emptying the property—a time of letting go and saying goodbye. It was definitely an emotional time for me. It was a period of grieving. My husband had died (22 years before my having bladder cancer), so I had nobody to help me do it. It took its toll.

Diagnosis of Bladder Cancer

I woke up in the middle of the night with severe abdominal pain. I tried to meditate it away. We went to Urgent Care, who recognized I was in trouble. They said, "We don't know what it is but you need to go to *(a hospital's)* emergency room." They discovered a mass in the bladder, as well as a cyst on my ovary. So, I knew that I was going to have surgery to get that thing out of there because it was attaching itself to other organs, and it hurt.

The diagnosis was out of the blue. I was really sort of non-plussed. I knew some awful things about bladder cancer and I just didn't want to go there. One thing that did strike me though, was that I realized, in retrospect, that as this tumor was growing, I was changing shape. I was bulging. I looked weird—it was disturbing. My kids were obviously scared; I'd never been sick before. Each of my sons said in his own way, "Mom, I love you. Whatever you decide to do, I support you", which was good to hear.

Treatment and Treatment Side Effects

I had surgery at 10 o'clock Monday morning and I was home at 10 o'clock Tuesday morning. The cyst on the ovary was benign, and the mass on the bladder was cancerous. *(The surgeon)* removed everything that he could find. It was minimally attached to the wall of the bladder. He also said that this type of bladder cancer is very aggressive and will probably come back. The surgery was done laparoscopically *(tube inserted through incision in abdomen to perform minor surgery)* so it wasn't bad at all. The major treatment side effect was constipation. I took the maximum amount of Tylenol for pain for only a week or 10 days post-surgery. I slept a lot.

Quality of Life During Treatment

Emotional State

I was so relieved that it wasn't ovarian cancer and that the bladder cancer had been contained. I had a hard time wrapping my head around the fact that I had cancer. It really took a while for that to settle in. I do not recall feeling absolutely devastated, which I think is probably in keeping with who I am. I was definitely concerned, but not terrified. But I was wondering what was next and how I was going to cope with it.

Relationships with Family, Friends, and Acquaintances

I have two children who live in the area, and a third one who lives outside of Chicago. I see the middle son, who has two daughters, and am most involved in their lives. We are close but not in each other's way. *(Since my move to Madison,)* I only know a few people out here. However, I do have a housemate, a companion, who took me to the ER. Since I healed quickly, I got back to exercising gently, did a lot of meditating, and a lot of deep breathing. I've also been doing gentle yoga ever since my husband's death. I found that helped. For me, that was very important.

Satisfaction with Medical Care During Treatment

That first day in the ER, they were keeping me comfortable with appropriate amounts of narcotics. I was in pain, yes, but not excruciating. It was manageable. The next day, the ER called me to see how I was doing. I had one of the best OB/GYN surgeons—oncologists and the urologist were excellent too. I certainly would recommend the surgeon. *(I got the information that I needed)* I think in part because I explained to them that I knew what they were talking about and if I didn't understand what they were saying I would ask them to clarify or to repeat it. Also, I told them that I had familiarity with the field and that I had been a hospice worker for a very long time. The relief on the look of the attending was wonderful.

When you are diagnosed with cancer you are traumatized. However, the oncologists didn't address any of the emotional components *(of having been treated for bladder cancer)*. I knew that would be true and I knew that was something I would have to address myself.

JACK KINKAID: *Bladder Cancer, disease stage not known, 85 years old, male, disease-free four years*

Life One Year Before Diagnosis

Before my diagnosis of bladder cancer, I felt fine; I had no worries. I had sciatica and spinal stenosis, but they don't really bother me that much. I just can't walk a lot anymore. A year before my diagnosis with bladder cancer I was diagnosed with COPD *(chronic obstructive pulmonary disease)*. I've had some skin cancers removed—nothing serious. Nothing was found a year ago. In the past I've had multiple operations: three hernias; an operation to remove a foot of my colon due to non-cancerous polyps that the doctors thought might grow and obstruct my colon; removal of a bunion on my foot; cataract surgeries on both eyes.

Diagnosis of Bladder Cancer

I noticed a darkening in my urine. My wife, who is a nurse, looked at it and said, "We better go see your doctor," my primary care physician. I went to see my doctor and he sees blood in my urine and a lump in my bladder. So my doctor sent me to a surgeon who decided that I would need to have an operation. I had no problem *(being told that I had bladder cancer)*. It is what it is, and you just get it taken care of. I was 81 years old at that time. Something's going to get me and I wasn't in pain. My primary care physician sent me to really good doctors. I trust him a lot.

Treatment and Treatment Side Effects

The surgeon removed the cancer. I asked him whether I needed further treatment. He said that with this type of bladder cancer, it was encapsulated *(enclosed as if in a capsule)* and there is no further treatment. All of a sudden I couldn't urinate anymore. They did a catheterization and the urine kept pouring out. The nurses kept changing *(an external)* bag *(which captured the urine)*. The surgeon decided to operate and after the surgery, I still couldn't urinate. I went home and went back to see my primary care physician. He put me in the hospital and shaved my prostate *(cut away some of the prostate to relieve pressure on the bladder)*, and that solved the problem. I was able to urinate and I've been fine ever since. There were no side effects from the surgery.

Quality of Life During Treatment

Relationships with Family, Friends, and Acquaintances

I have basically a 24/7 special duty nurse. I happened to marry her 53 years ago and she takes care of me. My children certainly got really concerned and very supportive. They were always in contact with me. My friends were also very supportive. I had all the love and help I needed.

Satisfaction with Medical Care During Treatment

I feel that I had good doctors, good hospitals, and good care. The nurses—it's amazing how good they are.

———————

AFTER TREATMENT AND THROUGH SURVIVORSHIP

NANCY S.: *Non-Muscle Invasive Bladder Cancer, Stage T1, High grade, 69 years old, female, disease-free two years*

Quality of Life After Treatment and Through Survivorship

Emotional State

The worst part is thinking there's never a time when you can think that bladder cancer is never going to come back. Every ache and pain you have, you think, "What is that? Could that be the cancer?" I feel fine up until the time when I have to have a test and then I get this anxiety thing. It's a week from tomorrow that I have a test. When you start out, it's every three months. Then after a while, it was every four months. I've been on an every-four-month schedule, and so I can kind of forget all about it for three months. Then I get this thing in the mail with my scheduled time and then I can just feel myself getting anxious. The thing is people say, "Well, don't you get less anxious because you're sort of in remission?" And I don't. I just get nervous as I did at the beginning, and maybe after ten years it will all ease up. *(My doctor)* told me the last time that we were going to go to six months and then after a little while, I'll go to one year and I'm not real happy about that. That seems like a long time between testing. But you never stop; you always get tested every year until you die.

Relationships with Family, Friends, and Acquaintances

I find myself gravitating to people who are struggling with something. In fact it's funny because there will be someone I'll meet who I really connected with, and then it turns out that that person is dealing with something, like diabetes. I think you find each other in that way.

Coping with Having Had Cancer

I started doing research, and as soon as I started doing that, I joined BCAN, the Bladder Cancer Advocacy Network, and some other forums, and started talking to other people. That really made a huge difference, because they started telling me about their experiences and their stories. I have met some great people. I found a woman who has bladder cancer through one of the BCAN forums, which is a bulletin board, where people go and write about anything and then people respond. Then you can go privately and become friends with people on this. She and I have the same doctor, and have gone to see him together. We are very, very close. She's been a great help to me and I to her. A fellowship of people who have the same problems, we all learn from each other. And aside from that, cancer just sucks.

The days that I decide that I'm going to be grateful for stuff are better days for me. It's too easy to get messed up, especially because all this stuff is going on and it's all scary and bad and if I can just take a moment and look at that blue sky up there, so pretty, that will help. *(Keep a)* gratitude journal, write down three things, or take three days of gratitude and just be aware. I keep talking about how lucky I am, and I do feel blessed, not in a religious way, but I am grateful for the people, the care I have, all of it.

Coping Needs That Were Unmet

A good bladder cancer support group would have been helpful.

Overall Impact of Having Had Cancer

Greatest Concerns

You're worrying about cancer a lot of the time. *(My greatest concern)* is that the cancer will come back. But I do feel like a very resilient person now. I'm proud of myself in that way, because the way I see it, you've got two choices: you can give up and whine a lot, or you can just say OK, that's the deal and I'm going to do whatever I can to help myself get through this. You never know what the ending is going to be. I'm very hopeful because I've now gone a long time with a lot of clear tests, and the longer you go the better, but there's no guarantee of anything. I'm just walking with that fear *(of the cancer coming back)*—just afraid of the unknown. I'm the kind of person who likes to know what is going to happen. I like things scheduled, and so it's very difficult to let go of that.

Advice

(Get the best medical center) that you can find, even if you have to travel. In the U.S. you can go to Sloan Kettering or MD Anderson or Mayo. You'll find a way to get there because that's where all the

research is going on, that's where the superstars are. I know a lot of people who put their heads in the sand; they don't want to know. But I would say knowledge is power and the more that you can learn, the less scary it is. Even with scary stuff there are options; you can do Option A, Option B—there is always a way that can make things less scary for yourself by learning.

MILLY H.: *Bladder Cancer, Stage II, 70 years old, female, disease-free four years*

Long-Term Treatment Side Effects

Exactly 13 months after my bladder was removed, I had a vaginal pro-lapse. I went to another urologist/gynecologist at *(the medical center)* who my doctor had recommended. He told me that all the staples holding the part of the vagina that remained had slipped and fallen and therefore my small intestine was literally falling out of my vagina *(enterocele)*. In January, 2015 I was back *(at the medical center)* having that repaired with lots of mesh. Exactly 13 months later it prolapsed again and my intestine fell again. In July of 2016. I was back at *(the medical center)* again to have that one repaired. But at least he was able to do it vaginally—they did not have to open my abdomen again, which I was very grateful for. Now I do pelvic floor exercises, thank-fully, everyday. I'm hoping this repair is a lifelong guarantee because that probably limited what I could do physically more than anything else. It's really hard to hide when you have an enterocele. It's really hard to do anything when part of your body is pushing out your vagina.

Quality of Life After Treatment and Through Survivorship

Emotional State

Fear of recurrence is not a prominent issue for me, but it is there a little more in the last six months because I had a really good friend whose bladder cancer came back after seven and a half years and she died. I have another friend right now whose bladder cancer has returned and *(as far as I know)* she has not died. She's gone silent *(though)*. I get no emails, I get no phone calls, so I'm very concerned that she has probably passed on. But it's not something I dwell on. I give this up to God and ask Him to take away my anxiety about it coming back. Why should you worry about what might happen in the future; why should you allow that to take away enjoying today? It just makes no sense to me.

Coping with Having Had Cancer

I think that I have to thank my mother for raising a strong-willed daughter. My mother was a Depression-era baby who was taught that the only role women had in life was to stay home and raise children. But she raised my sister and I to want more than that and she raised us to be strong. I really thank my mother for making me a strong person because I think I get it from her. Even though she wasn't around for any of this, I still felt like she was there for me. I constantly heard from my family, "You just better not give up, Mom; you better fight this." I had it pretty much set in my head that I wasn't going to give up, at least not at that point anyway.

I was usually able to pull out of the depressions with the support I had and I think with God's help. The Bladder Cancer Advocacy Network (BCAN) Inspire Group *(online website for patients)* was amazing. There were actually people I had never met before the year I was in the hospital. If they lived anywhere near me, they came to visit me. I used to think the support I had there from friends and family, and the wonderful staff there, kept me from being an emotional wreck, because I could have been an emotional wreck.

Religion

I have not joined a church, but I have considered it. I live in a small rural area where most of the churches have five or six members.

That's not something I'm looking for. It's like I'm in church when I go out hiking and look at everything God has made for us to enjoy. I do bring the bible more often. I can't say it's a daily occurrence because it's not. I do pray every day, more to thank God than anything else. I'm still grappling with my religious beliefs and yeah, it's probably going to be a lifelong process grappling with my religious beliefs.

Coping Needs That Were Not Met

My family took turns staying with me and helping me during chemo. After surgery it would have been helpful for my family to be around, but since they all lived so far away it just wasn't possible. I could have asked my friends to visit more often, but I felt they had done so much for me for months. I just read many hours a day while recovering from surgery. Living in a rural area is wonderful, but it can be lonely. Once I was able to get back to my crafts and my exercise I was fine.

Overall Impact of Having Had Cancer

I think it changed my whole outlook on life. I think it made me realize what joy I have around me every day. It has made me thankful for all the resources that I have available to me. I am more thankful for my family. I'm thankful every morning when I wake up. It's not an effort to find joy every day; the joy is just there. It's recognizing that life has become so much easier. You go from one day when you're pretty sure you're about to die, and then you realize you're not. Then you're so thankful that you've got all this time that could have ended four years ago, that it could still end tomorrow—who knows? So find the joy everyday.

When I realized how giving people were to me, some of whom were virtual strangers, some of them were people I'd known a long time, who gave their time and their resources to help me get through this. It gave me a new mindset of looking out at the world and finding ways to be of help to people. I think that I'm less selfish now. Before, I was so worried about keeping my financial resources for me, being stingy, not wanting to give out anything to anybody. I find myself a much more giving person now.

(My family is) closer now than it was prior. A lot of it had to do with where everybody lived. The two older boys (sons) were always best friends, but geographically they weren't close. They got closer after my cancer diagnosis because they were together more often— they made an effort to be at my home. We've had several family reunions since then because I decided I can't take my money with me. Go and spend it on something important. So we've got a family reunion in Mexico. We've made a concerted effort to get all members of the family together, which has brought them both closer. I think I developed more diverse friendships with a lot people that I would never have known. I can't think of anybody that dropped out, of anybody that was made uncomfortable.

Greatest Concerns

I think of the consequences of aging—whether I'm going to be able to take care of myself, do the things I need to do to stay in my home by myself. I think about that, more often than I think about what the cancer has done to me. Will my arthritis and my hands get so bad that I couldn't cut the holes out of the external bag from my bladder? Little things like that concern me.

Advice

Put yourself out there, ask for help and support, don't try to hide what you think might be an embarrassing form of cancer. There are a lot of people that think bladder cancer shouldn't be talked about. It should be. Talk about it, ask for help, find a support group. If you're religious, get people praying for you. If you're not religious, fine, get people to send you good thoughts.

JOE C.: *Bladder Cancer, Stage IV, 72 years old, male, disease-free two years*

Long-Term Treatment Side Effects

The biggest physical issue I have now is that my bladder will get full after about 4.5–5 hours. I need to set the clock for the middle of the night, each night, and get up and go relieve myself.

Quality of Life After Treatment and Through Survivorship

Emotional State

When I really began to prepare for the CT scan a couple of days before it happens, then that's at the point where I start thinking about it. I wouldn't say I dread it, but it's on my mind, "Gosh, I hope they wouldn't find anything." I'm not really thinking they will, but it's always in the back of my mind, "What if they do?"

Sexual Life

I haven't really recovered from the surgery. I can't sustain any useful erections. The urge is there, but it's just not going to happen. My wife had some of her own gynecological issues over this year, so she's not eager for intercourse. We are still physically intimate and enjoy each other physically, but full intercourse just doesn't happen.

Regaining and/or Changing One's Life

I've been active for my whole life. To me, being able to move and able to exercise is something that I've always found comfort in and enjoyment from. Within six weeks after I left the hospital I was starting to go back to the gym and do some really mild exercises. My wife and I were both worried about possible incontinence issues, but I put on diapers. The biggest change in terms of what my wife and I do is we haven't traveled overseas since the surgery. We used to travel widely in Central American and Latin American countries. I think we're both at an age when each of us feel more secure if we were not doing the kind of adventure travels that we used to do, which are far away from any kind of medical emergency situations. *(However, there were)* a lot of physical things that I loved to do that I can't do anymore. We used to play lots of beach volleyball, lots of tennis, and I was a collegiate athlete. I loved high-jumping. I used to go to the ocean and body surf. I'm older now and I just can't or don't want to do those things because I don't trust myself physically.

I fell back into normal interactions with everybody pretty quickly. I don't think I took any trauma away from the experience. I don't think I feel more vulnerable. I think having a network of family and friends have been the biggest thing. A really good friend of mine referred me to another friend of his who had a neobladder. Dealing with both of these guys gave me a good preview of what might be the future or what would be my experience. I think it was invaluable to me in terms of making my choices and getting a grasp on it. Without having spoken to these guys on a face-to-face basis, it would have been much more difficult.

Satisfaction with Medical Care after Treatment and Through Survivorship

I do get concerned *(when there are mild signs of a problem)*. Luckily, my local urologist has a pretty open communication. I can email him anytime I want. For example, a couple of times I've had minor amounts of blood in my urine. I call him, email him, and then we get in touch. He was very soothing. He says, "That's something in my experience that just happens sometimes and it might be something you ate or that you had some unusual physical activity. If it doesn't have any other symptoms without fever or any other kinds of symptomatic display, then it's nothing you need to be concerned about."

Overall Impact of Having Had Cancer

I'm probably more interested in reaching out to people I used to know or know now, and see what I can do to help them in their lives. I'm a little more externally directed probably because of the kindness that people showed me when I was having my most difficult times. The things that I responded to most often are people who have just been diagnosed and are in a total panic. I'm trying to tell them that it's possible that you can do well. You can stand more than you think you can stand in terms of the hardships involved. I just make people aware that it's really tough. Things can turn out well and it's not a reason to be super despairing until things turn out worse.

I tried to do some outreach online and personally, with people who are facing the same situation. I talked to a couple of people who had experienced cystectomies and just speaking to those people really helped me to make decisions and to gain insight into what their situation was going be. I met with a couple of people who live nearby and were faced with a radical cystectomy. I just talked to them informally and said this has been my experience, and answer questions and try to reassure them that if all goes well and life goes on, you'll be fine.

Greatest Concerns

The greatest concern is just trying to keep in good physical condition, and as long as I can, be active. I think that's key to keep my metabolism and my whole body intact. I think the fear would be that there's some mechanical failure with the neobladder. I wouldn't want to have to be catheterizing myself all the time *(which might require)* another big surgery to correct things. It's not something that I dwell on. Honestly, I'm just happy to be alive and functional every day.

Advice

A great deal of the positive *(medical)* outcome had to do with acting early and quickly, and having very, very good experts and treatment from the get-go. I feel like all of the urologists that I dealt with were highly informed and very competent, who networked with other doctors constantly to keep themselves informed. If your urologist is not a bladder cancer specialist, they sometimes are out of touch with what are the latest protocols and what really ought to be done or what's best practice at any given point. I think people should look for second opinions and go to a National Cancer Institute hospital and seek out people who treat bladder cancer every day, rather than a generalized urologist.

It does no good at all to dread and create fears that are unwarranted. It calls for a lot of determination, both emotionally and physically. But, the most destructive thing that you can do, in my mind, is dreading and despairing, to lose hope *(in having)* a positive outcome.

MIKE S.: *Bladder Cancer, Stage T1, 73 years old, male, disease-free one year*

Quality of Life after Treatment and Through Survivorship

Emotional State

This was a quiet killer; it was an assassin. There was no warning, no pain, no discomfort, no anything. Now, *(after all treatment,)* there's no physical ailment, no discomfort. Because I'm walking four miles a day, I'm lifting the 10-pound weights, I'm doing my sit-ups, I'm back. After a year, my doctor said that everything showed up perfect. I'm one of the lucky ones that became a survivor. I don't take any day or any second *(for granted)* anymore.

Coping with Having Had Cancer

My motivation was my four year old granddaughter. I wanted to see her grow up.

Overall Impact of Having Had Cancer

Positive Effects

I'm always a positive person. I had a wonderful mother and father, I married well, delight in my daughters, the life, everything I've done, teaching, my vocation. But since *(having had cancer)*, I just realized I don't take anything for granted anymore, such as the little things, the simple things. I always felt I was a nice person, but now I'm much nicer. Now I'm no more in a rush. I go meet someone— nothing is more important than talking to a person. There was one fellow from Maine that was going to go through the same thing as me. He wanted to hear about *(having bladder cancer)* from a civilian point of view. He asked me to speak to him. So, I got on the phone and spoke to him and told him exactly what he's going to go through. I just wanted to be there. I want to be there for everybody. I just want to enjoy every second of every day.

Greatest Concern

My greatest concern is that the cancer will come back.

Advice

Once it's diagnosed and it's there, then stop feeling sorry for yourself and attack it. Go for it with everything you have. Listen to what the doctors say, follow directions, stay positive, and hope that everything works out well.

SHARRON O.: *Bladder Cancer, Stage IV, 76 years old, female, disease-free one year*

Long-Term Treatment Effects

I did have to wear a dress one day and it was really a difficult thing because I was like, "OK, if I get really big pantyhose, they won't stay up *(because of the external bag)*, and if I get small ones, they will put pressure on the stoma because it does actually stick out a half-to three quarters of an inch. Since it doesn't have any nerves, you don't feel anything. But if you push hard enough on it, there's a sensation inside that's not painful, but it is uncomfortable. That's one issue that I probably still need to resolve if I ever decided I want to wear a dress again. But generally, I wear pants, generally jeans, and it doesn't show. Most people if they know, they forget and if they don't know, they don't have any clue.

Quality of Life After Treatment and Through Survivorship

Emotional State

I was terrified that *(the bladder cancer)* was going to come back and that I would have chemo. *(When asked whether the fear of recurrence was really the fear of chemo, I said)* "Yes." Subconsciously, I avoided other cancer patients because I didn't want to make my having had cancer my whole life.

Non-Cancer Stresses

(Six months before my diagnosis of bladder cancer), I tripped over the cement curb and shattered my elbow and shoulder. My therapy for recovery from the elbow surgery was very long and intense, which was temporarily interrupted due to having bladder cancer surgery. *(A month)* after the bladder cancer surgery I underwent surgery for a complete total reverse shoulder replacement. At this point in time,

I am seeing much more mobility throughout my entire body. Still probably a year to go before my shoulder and arm are 90% or better. The muscles that had been immobile due to the shoulder dislocation have loosened, and my cancer incision areas now feel much better. I get more frustrated with what I can't do because of my arm. I understand that this makes it difficult because I actually have two processes going on at the same time. But I get real frustrated because I go to reach for something and my arm doesn't work. My body works fine, except for my arm.

Coping with Having Had Cancer

The best thing that helped me cope through most of my life when *(I'm)* in sheer and absolute panic is, "Stop and take a deep breath, and we'll go on from here", which is I think what got me through a lot of the tough times. I remember laying back on the table *(in the surgery room)* going into 12 hours of surgery for cancer, and saying to myself, "Just take a deep breath and let it go."

I don't panic very easily. I don't take stupid chances. I've always been very, very calculating on what I did before I did it, and as a result, I've done more things than probably most people have ever dreamed of. It's not like, "If I don't make it out of surgery, I will have missed so much." I've got great kids, great grandchildren. I've got five incredibly wonderful, great-grandsons. Why would I feel like I missed anything? It's kind of, "OK, if that's going to happen, it's going to happen; but in the meantime, I'm just going to do what I do day-to-day." That seems to have worked out well. I want to live every day the best I can. I'm not doomsday at all.

Biofeedback

(About 10 years ago) my ex-husband asked me to help him with an experiment he was doing, "biofeedback training." I spent probably six months being trained on how to block out what I didn't want to

think about and to focus on either going blank or putting my brain someplace where I wanted it to be. For me, it works better to go blank more than anything else. It's the same thing I did the morning of the cancer surgery. I knew that my son and my friend were there and that they were very stressed, and I just chose to put my brain someplace else.

Overall Impact of Having Had Cancer

Negative and Positive Effects

I find that I am much more willing to sit and do nothing, and I'm OK with it more than I used to be. But that's about the only thing I can think of that's positive. *(However)*, I guess it would be nicer not to have a bag on the side of my body. But it's not a big deal that I get worked up about.

Greatest Concerns

I prefer "focus" to "concern," and my focus is to keep getting through this one day at a time. I've had a great run so far—haven't had anything left on my "bucket list" *(achievements to have in a lifetime)*, other than to create a new "bucket list."

Advice

If a person has the option and wherewithal to purchase PPO *(Preferred Provider Organization)* insurance for themselves, it is worth the investment, even if it means a sacrifice. If there is something really, really wrong with you, the ability to have the PPO coverage *(greater size of the plan network, ability to see specialists, coverage for out of network services)* and to go to *(an excellent medical center)*, makes such a difference, compared to going through the HMO process, which is literally "you take what you can get."

SCOTT: *Bladder Cancer, Early Stage, 79 years old, male, disease-free one year*

Quality of Life after Treatment and Through Survivorship

Relationships with Family, Friends, and Acquaintances

(My brother and I) communicate far more often than we did before. My other brother is supportive but in a much more distant way. When we talk, he's always saying, "How're you doing?" *(My son-in-law)* always says, "If you want to talk about anything, give me a call." My relationship with my friends might have gotten a bit better. A few times I had to be dependent on them for transportation assistance, which they were happy to provide. There's a woman who I know who has had cancer after I had cancer. Before that, we were always, "Hi, how are you doing?" Her relationship with me has changed completely because we sit down and talk about life now.

Social Life

I had to miss a couple of functions because of the bleeding from the wound in my stomach. That didn't bother me much.

Financial Problems

(After I was terminated from my job), I was actively looking for a job until *(I got this wound in my stomach)*. Then I had to stop because I couldn't go to an employer and say, "Let me go to work for you, but I have to be home every day to get a dressing change *(from the visiting nurse for the stomach wound)*." *(Before I was terminated)*, I went out to dinner with my family once or twice a month. I never worried about *(being able to pay for the meal)*. I am now in a position where I really worry about it. We had a very limited Christmas this year. This past year, we haven't been away on vacation, and *(I'm more limited in being able to)* entertain my grandkids, all primarily because of my financial status.

Other Non-Cancer Medical Problems

I got up and am standing in the kitchen, and I feel something warm running down my leg. I found that I had a hole in my stomach and that fluid was coming out of there. The urology surgeon just kind of dismissed me. He was sure the problem was due to a fistula and had nothing to do with his surgery. So he didn't want to deal with it. He pushed me off to *(another doctor)* who was "much more of a fistula expert." *(After the procedure concerning the fistula was done)*, I now have a hole in my belly and it has to heal from the inside out. I had a nurse come to the house every day to change the dressing and repack the wound, but it's still open and draining every day. I'm still dealing with packing *(the hole so that the fluid doesn't come out)* everyday. I find it to be a real nuisance that I have to be available when the visiting nurse is available to have this thing repacked every day. But once this is healed, hopefully I'm done. It's become one thing *(medical problem)* after another.

Other than this wound, I don't have any real physical problems that constrain me in any way. My cardiac problems, GI problems and kidney problems *(that I had during treatment)* are OK.

Coping with Having Had Cancer

The external pouch is there and it's relatively easy to take care of. I don't have a problem doing it myself. It's uncomfortable, but at the same time, it's part of me now.

(My girlfriend) knows me. She also knows cancer as well, if not better than some doctors that she works with. The team behind her who *(served as)* my second opinion through all of this, was invaluable. The relationship between me and my youngest brother got better as well. He really stepped up.

Overall Impact of Having Had Cancer

Positive Effect

People *(who have cancer)* listen now *(to what I have to say)* because they know I have gone through it.

Greatest Concerns

Financial problems are the biggest concern I have at the moment. The financial impact *(of having been fired from my job due to my having cancer)* has been unbelievable.

Advice

Number 1—Do anything and everything you can to take care of the cancer. Number 2—Change your lifestyle to adapt to whatever treatment plan is presented to you. Number 3—Give whatever medical options you're given as much thought as you can, but don't waste a lot of time, because cancer doesn't. Number 4—If you have any kind of a support team from family and friends, don't be afraid to use them.

PAULINE N.: *Bladder Cancer, Stage IV, 81 years old, female, disease-free one year*

Long-Term Treatment Effects

It has been two years *(since the surgery)*. I'm still having problems with the colostomy *(external pouch)*, but it's tolerable. I put it on myself. It's a pain in the neck, but that's the best you can do. That's what you have to do. It doesn't limit me with being with my friends.

Quality of Life after Treatment and Through Survivorship

Emotional State

I have a CT scan every three months. I feel like I live three months at a time, because the next time I have the CT scan, *(it could show that the tumor had started growing)*. Your life is on hold. You live while you're alive and you make basically no plans for the future, which when you're 80 years old, you don't make plans for the future anyway. Some people even at 80 have a lot of energy. I'm not one of those people. The type of illness I have has really put me down, in every aspect of my life. Sometimes I think, when there's a tragedy in the family, a tragedy like this cancer, maybe it's better that that person dies. I think people go through a tragedy once or that they try to put it away. It's not fair for the people who are alive to be hanging around when you're almost dead. I feel like there's not much *(left in life)* for me. I love to be loved. I want to look nice. I want to travel. That's what I love. I would love to be young again and not at the end of my life.

Regaining and/or Changing One's Life

In my life I always wanted not to be dirt poor. I wanted to do everything I could to advance myself and to have enough. I wanted to be self-sufficient, and to have something and to give something to my kids. This was very important to me. What I mostly wanted was to be independent. Being a nurse, I was able to do that. I'm so thankful that I've been able to take care of the *(nursing home residents)* and I promised that I would always make sure that nothing happens to them, that nobody will mistreat them.

I can still go to my nursing home *(where I was the director)* and the people wait for me there. I had a very close relationship with the patients in the nursing home. They know me and they miss me. They pull a chair up and tell me to sit down. It's all a support group from those people. I always became very close with their families. It was emotionally very satisfying because not only did I like the elderly people, but I also loved their families, and they loved coming to my place. A lot of times, even after *(their parent)* passed away, their *(son/daughter)* would still come. That makes me very happy.

But I had to get a director of nurses, which I used to be. I could be involved in the nursing home if I really want to. The nice thing about it is that I don't have to be. If I don't feel good or I don't feel like going, I don't have to. Although we have a director of nurses, she calls me to find out what would I do in a case like that. Nothing like an old wolf. The older you are, the more experienced you are, the more you acquire more knowledge about how to treat people, and what's important and what not to worry about. I'm still involved in that.

Functioning

My housekeeper comes three days each week. *(In addition to her cleaning the house)*, we go grocery shopping and shopping for clothes. She's a wonderful person. I don't need any more help than that because I can do a lot of things for myself.

Relationships with Family, Friends, and Acquaintances

My kids—they're very, very, very supportive. I don't need any help from my children *(to do housekeeping)*. I have a housekeeper. The only thing that I need from my children is just to talk to them, to come over and visit. One of my children is now in charge of the nursing home. There has been some animosity from my other children. They want to say how to run *(the nursing home)*. You cannot run a business with five people *(my children and me)*. There has to be the boss. My kids suffered so much *(due to my having cancer)*. They have gone through the shock of losing me. I think they buried me already. It's not all of my children, just a couple of them. The whole thing is about money. My kids are not young kids anymore. I have a son who's going to be 60. How long are they going to wait for their inheritance? I think that a couple of them want to sell the nursing home and divide the money. Some of them want to keep it. As long as I'm alive, I'm in charge.

A lot of my friends have passed away. I'm not depressed because of that, because I know that that's the way it is. But some of my friends are still alive, and you just enjoy the little visits you have with them. However, I'm a very private person. I'm talking to you *(the interviewer)* and telling you that, but this is something I would not share with friends. First of all, I don't want to hear them say, "You poor thing." Second of all, if people don't understand you, then they judge you. Even when they say, "I understand how it is," they don't understand. They don't know anything at all.

Non-Cancer Medical Problems

I didn't take my blood thinner for four days that I was supposed to be taking it, and I had a stroke. That is the thing that has incapacitated me more than the cancer. My stroke is not a real bad one. I have a hard time walking—I have to use a walker. *(The stroke also)* incapacitated me by affecting my eyes. I couldn't see for a couple months.

Coping Needs That Were Not Met

I am getting to the point to where I would really like to speak or to meet some other people that have the same problem, somebody who's like me, to talk about how they're coping and what they are doing with their life.

Overall Impact of Having Had Cancer

Advice

Be around people, around your friends. You don't have to tell them what you have. Try to feel as normal as possible. If you don't have pain or anything, just live your life, as God would provide it for you. Do the best you can.

TERRY TUPPER: *Bladder Cancer, Stage I, Grade 4, 85 years old, female, disease-free one year*

Quality of Life after Treatment and Through Survivorship

Emotional State

I think that the piece that was scary and continues to be scary was that this is a very aggressive form of bladder cancer that comes back. Every little ache, every little twitch, every little something that you've never had before, suddenly becomes cancer. The longer out you get, statistically it is less likely to come back. So, I am now a year and three months out, with no evidence of disease. The urological oncologist said, "Let's wait for six months *(for the next scan and cystoscopy)*, so that if there is something growing there we will be able to see it." His point obviously being that it is an aggressive form of bladder cancer. It takes time for it to be visible so that we can see those cells. I felt anxious two weeks ahead of time *(of the scan or cystoscopy)*. Then it really peaked three to five days before the appointment, and my anxiety goes through the roof. Then afterwards you get to see you didn't have to be so anxious.

Relationships with Family, Friends, and Acquaintances

My sons called, they checked in on me. They kept saying, "I love you, Mom" and "How is it going?" Two of my sons are pretty monosyllabic, so to get that much emotional response out of them, even if it's a text or email, or a phone call, I felt their presence, and that's what matters.

(People who have not experienced having cancer and the fear of it recurring) just don't understand that even though statistically the odds may be in your favor *(of the cancer not coming back)*, they don't "get it"—that the glass can be half full or half empty. They don't have a clue. Because of that, I have a tendency to keep it to myself. It is very isolating, a very lonely place. I do not share with *(new members at the support group at Gilda's Club)* that I am a survivor. My reactions have been validated by people describing the same phenomena. *(However)*, during a support group at Gilda's Club, even though I had to contain myself, I got vicarious support from them *(by listening to what members of the group said)*.

Religion/Spirituality

I don't know what's out there, but I know that there is more out there than what's here. I feel deeply connected with something and that something is inside me that I call "the little one," the one I can love.

Prior Medical and Non-Medical Stresses

When I was very, very young, my father emotionally and sexually abused me, using inappropriate sexual behavior. My sister died when she was 22 years old due to a gas heater, which wasn't installed properly. She woke up to a room full of gas and couldn't get the window open fast enough. My daughter committed suicide when she was 20 years old. She was an adopted child, probably had fetal alcohol syndrome, and had a borderline personality. She just decided that her life was miserable.

When one has gone through certain events (*father's sexual and emotional abuse*), you get through them—you don't get over them. Getting through this cancer enabled me to go back (*in time*), revisit these events and to let go somehow, to be kinder to myself. I was so young that it just influenced so much of one's being. I think having cancer was almost like a wake-up call. "Come on, you have got work to do here before you can go off to wherever you are going." So, from that point of view I think it gave me the strength to do that.

Coping with Having Had Cancer

I think what does help me cope is not letting myself perseverate on it (*having had cancer*), which isn't to say that I don't at times get really anxious about that. I say, "OK, you know what else this is about? It's part of my aging process." I am in the last chapter of my life, however many more years. I am not afraid of being dead. I am concerned about how I die.

What also helps when I am feeling blue and under a cloud, is getting out and engaging in the world. And whether it's out digging in my garden which I love, going for a walk, or playing my clarinet, or working with people, or being in a caregiver, caring, or therapeutic role. After my husband died, I was a grief counselor at Grace Hospice as a volunteer for 12 years. After Grace Hospice, I began working at Gilda's Club in 2009 as a facilitator in groups, both for people who have cancer and for caretakers. It wasn't particularly cancer that drew me, it was working with folks who could benefit from mutual support. With folks at Gilda's Club, that's what nourishes my soul so much.

I do have a close friend who has had breast cancer and, most recently, endometrial cancer. She and I get together twice a month and we are able to share our stories, because we each "get it" *(understand how cancer has affected our lives).* That has been a very helpful relationship and we appreciate each other and tell each other that. It's not a one-sided thing—it's mutual. It's those bonds that are so critical.

Coping Needs That Were Unmet

I think it's just my position as a facilitator at Gilda's Club and being with people who "get it," and who are speaking to me unwittingly, that I could have used being in a support group. But there is no support group for this cancer. Support groups should definitely be part of hospitals' provision of psychosocial services for cancer patients. I know they're short-staffed and they don't have it in their budget, but they definitely need to have them so that you don't have to face cancer alone.

Overall Impact of Having Had Cancer

Negative and Positive Effects

Having had cancer is a gift in terms of my having coped with it as best as I could. From a negative point of view, "Who needs cancer?" It does occupy my mind. Once you are diagnosed with cancer, you are changed.

Greatest Concerns

Probably, given my age, my greatest concern is getting rid of some more stuff *(in my home)* so my kids don't have to declutter, so as not to be a burden to them. Recently, I have already taken steps about a green burial *(does not slow down the body's decomposition, in order to have less impact on the earth)*. I am taking care of things like that. Each of my kids thanked me for doing this so that they don't have to figure out what it was that I wanted. I'm getting the little tasks done—accepting what is coming and being okay with it.

Advice

Be kind to yourself; have patience with yourself. You are not a bad person because you have cancer. Try to keep it in perspective and get the kind of help you need.

JACK KINKAID: *Bladder Cancer, disease stage not known, 85 years old, male, disease-free four years*

Quality of Life after Treatment and Through Survivorship

Emotional State

I've never thought that in any of the medical problems I've had over the years that I was going to die. I'm just the type of person who doesn't get upset about these things. My wife goes on the computer and she gets all the information *(I need)* and explains everything to me. You have a problem, you take care of it. Maybe I'm just fortunate that I didn't get upset by this. But it doesn't really do you any good if you get upset. I just take it in stride.

Regaining and/or Changing One's Life

Once they let me out of the hospital, it took probably several months to recover. I couldn't go play golf or anything for a while, until three months later. After that, I was pretty well on my way. Walking is not a problem until I've walked a few blocks and then my left leg starts getting a little numb. When I can just sit down and rest for a few minutes I'm fine again. The only thing I won't be able to do anymore is going on any long trips, because I really can't do a lot of walking.

Relationships with Family, Friends, and Acquaintances

I'm the last one left in my family. I was the youngest and now I've lived longer than anybody. I expected it. It's not traumatic—people are going to die. I'm going to die someday. I'm originally from South Jersey *(section of New Jersey)*, and only two of my friends who I grew up with are still alive. I have one couple here. We go out to dinner with them once a week, and that's it. But it's nice.

Coping with Having Had Cancer

I made up my mind. I would do what I could do, while I can do it. When I couldn't do it anymore, I'm finished. I think religion probably *(helped me deal with having had bladder cancer)*. My wife and I are both Catholic and we go to church every Sunday, even when we're away.

Overall Impact of Having Had Cancer

Negative and Positive Effects

There were absolutely no negative or positive changes in my life because I had cancer.

Greatest Concerns

The only thing I'm concerned about is making sure that my wife has a life that is outside of our life. Hopefully, I will die before she does. She is a really good person. She has a life of her own now, besides ours, which is what I want. When I go, I want her to still have friends.

Advice

Make sure you get good doctors and a totally good hospital. Don't get too upset about having cancer. I don't know how you could control that, but getting upset doesn't do you any good. In fact, it may do you harm. Lean on your loved ones. It really helps to have people supporting you. You have to have people who you can really joke around with, and talk with, and have a good time. I have that with my golfing buddies and my neighbors and friends here. If you don't have anybody, you might be in serious trouble.

Chapter 2

Older Survivors of Colorectal Cancer

As 140,250 colorectal cancer patients were diagnosed in 2018, colorectal cancer became the fourth largest type of cancer when compared to all other cancer diagnoses in the United States. Half of patients diagnosed with colon cancer were diagnosed when 65 years old or older (56.3%). The survival rate of five years or more is roughly three-quarters of colorectal cancer patients who are 65 years old or older (National Cancer Institute, SEER Cancer Stat Facts).

Several studies have been done that place a light on several important issues that help to describe and understand the quality of life of colorectal cancer survivors. A nationwide study was done in Australia concerning the quality of life and life satisfaction of 1,966 colorectal cancer survivors over a five-year period (Dunn et al. 2013). Those survivors whose quality of life continued to be excellent or who had a good quality of life over time was reported by three-quarters of the group (73.3%). However, 19.2% reported that their quality of life was always low, beginning soon after their diagnosis, and persisting at a low level over the following five years. If you take the number of those reporting a low quality of life, 255,760 patients would be in that low quality of life category that would persist over five years after they were diagnosed.

On the other side of the coin, Dr. Jansen (Jansen et al. 2011) did a study of the positive effects of having had cancer in 483 colorectal cancer patients in Germany. Ninety percent of the sample was 60 years old or older. Sixty-four percent of patients reported that there were positive consequences of having had cancer, with 46% reporting positive changes in their view of life, relationships with their family and friends, and how they felt about themselves. It may come as a surprise to some of the readers of the book that something positive can come out of having had cancer, in addition, of course, to becoming a survivor, in remission or free of disease. When you read the interviews of colorectal cancer survivors you will see that some of these survivors talk about *both* the negative and positive effects of having had cancer.

———

INTO AND THROUGH TREATMENT

JIM M.: *Colorectal Cancer, Stage IV, 68 years old, male, disease-free one year*

Life One Year Before Diagnosis

Before I was diagnosed *(with colorectal cancer)* *, I thought that everything was going pretty good in my life. We're really close to our kids. It's just wonderful that our kids love being with us—we love being with them. My grandson was born two months before I went into the emergency room. We were very happy that our family was growing. Family life was great. I didn't have any issues there. I was still working and that was going fine. I was jogging *(running)* all the time. I was also a bike rider. I was playing golf with my kids, so I was very active. Everything seemed to be going good. The only *(medical problem)* I was having was gout flare-ups, and I would get them maybe every nine months to a year. It lasted for a couple of weeks and it was very painful. Through the years of mainly Catholic schooling, we accumulated a number of friends. We get together with probably half a dozen friends from the church and from the school. We have a pretty much active social life. We've also hooked up with other musicians of our age. Music is really a big part of our lives.

---

* *Italicized (slanted) typing is used in parentheses when quoting participants to complete their sentences, in order to make the quotes clearer.*

Even though I didn't go to a doctor *(for 45 years)* and felt really good, I felt that somehow, sometime, that is all going to end, which it did. I did notice that I wasn't able to run as far or as fast as I normally could and I attributed it to getting older. About a month before *(I was diagnosed)* I started losing my appetite and food didn't taste right.

So at that point in time I knew something was wrong. I was afraid of going to the doctor, that I was going to find out that something was horribly wrong.

Diagnosis of Colorectal Cancer

I didn't know if it's my wife or if it was God or what, but I was never afraid of any of the diagnoses when they told me that I had Stage IV cancer. It wasn't like: "Oh, my God, this is horrible." I knew that it was bad, but at that point, I sort of put it in the hands of my doctors and God, in terms of what was going to happen from that point on.

At first it's like who do you tell? And I figured I had to tell everybody. It was hard to tell, but after I told one person, it just became easier and easier to tell people what I had, what I was going through. I think that can help people. It might make the person on the receiving end of the news a little uncomfortable, but I think it's good for the cancer patient. I think ultimately it helps people that you're telling them *(of having cancer)* because then they realize they can talk to you about your treatment and they aren't stepping on eggshells. It seems like when you disclose what you have, people are there to help you.

Treatment and Treatment Side Effects

(Before surgery) I was in more and more pain. Not much worked *(to reduce the pain)*. I had to urinate more frequently, which made it even more painful. It got down to where I could only sleep for 45 minutes at a time and I would wake up and have to pee, and it would take me about 15 to 20 minutes to get back to sleep.

Unfortunately I had to wait two months before I had all the authorizations for the surgery. At that time I was in a lot of pain and discomfort. It would have helped if that process could have been quicker. In addition, at this time leading up to the surgery, I had problems in being able to sleep and really having any sort of quality of life. It just crumbled. My oncologist did tell me that the use of cannabis *(marijuana)* could help. I did use a lot of cannabis leading up to my surgery, and then some after my surgery. I think cannabis helped relieve the anxiety of the upcoming surgery. So, going into the surgery, I really didn't have any anxiety or fear of the surgery.

The major surgery was to remove the tumor in my colon. The cancer had destroyed my bladder, so they removed the bladder and the prostate. I was having more issues with my bladder than with my colon. My urologist gave me three choices: I could have the neo-bladder surgery where they removed my bladder *(and created a new bladder from the small intestine)*, or the Indiana pouch *(internal storage of urine after the bladder is removed, and drained by using a tube attached to the outside of the body, several times a day)*, or the external pouch *(urine flows to an external pouch though an opening in the wall of the stomach)*. I chose the external pouch because I wanted to sleep. I knew that there was going to be the least amount of problems with it. It doesn't bother me that much. I think that if I were younger I probably would have gone for the neobladder so I would look normal. I think that it bothers my wife a little bit. She doesn't really like looking at my stoma. She doesn't like it when I have to change my bag. She'd rather be in the other room and not watch. It doesn't bother me when I'm out and I have to empty my bag. I just go into the public restrooms and step up to the urinal. Instead of unzipping my pants, I pull my bag out and empty it into the urinal.

My stomach started giving me more problems. I was more nauseated. So, they did a CT scan on me and then the next day they did a scope of my stomach, found out that I had a bleeding ulcer from some of the medication that I was taking for the swelling of my foot. They gave me a pill, Protonix. That worked immediately.

It was sort of an up-and-down period, where before the surgery I would feel a lot of discomfort and pain. Then right after the surgery, I got better. "OK, you're better; now you are well enough to go into the chemo to destroy any cancer cells." But then also, it is wreaking havoc on other parts of the body. I think the worst thing about the chemo was the loss of appetite and just how horrible food tasted. The other big thing from the chemo was it just makes you weak. It just saps all of your energy out of you. The last rounds of chemo I wasn't as nauseated as I was during the middle *(rounds of chemo)*, but it was just making me weaker and weaker. The oncology nurses would always ask me: "Do you feel a tingling in your fingers or toes?" I didn't have that until the 11th round of chemo, and I didn't understand what it was. They didn't tell me what it was, but it was neuropathy.

When they sent me home after surgery or after some of the procedures, *(they would give me)* a heavy duty *(medication)* like oxycodone *(pain killer)*. It gave me anxiety and it gave me nightmares. My primary care doctor prescribed some other *(pain)* medications. Tramadol is one. It's more potent than Tylenol but not quite so potent as oxycodone and other opioids. That helped. I did use marijuana—it helped me sleep. It took away a little bit of the pain.

Quality of Life During Treatment

Emotional State

I knew that what I had was bad, but in my mind, I'm not going to let it totally control my life. I always felt that tomorrow might be better, or the next day might be better. So, even if I was in a lot of pain and discomfort, I just kept thinking that things would get better. I still need some sort of control in my life. I always felt that I had that. Whenever I was going downhill quickly, my wife I think thought I was going to die. I never really felt that way. I felt that if I can make it through the day, there is tomorrow. If I can do it again the next day, then I can get through this. I never knew when I would feel good. For about a year I missed all the birthday gatherings. I missed the christening of my grandson, Christmas, Thanksgiving—all the holidays.

Relationships with Family, Friends, and Acquaintances

(My wife) doesn't break down very easily, although I know that it does affect her—hearing bad news. My wife was with me for every doctor's appointment. She's really been my strength. I think that everybody going through cancer needs a very strong caregiver. If your caregiver is weak, it's just going to bring you down. I think that a strong care-giver can make such a big difference in the way you go though the journey of having cancer. I think our relationship has probably got-ten stronger. I really thank her for being by my side. There have been times where I was in a lot of pain and I knew it was really hard on my wife. She didn't break down and cry, she didn't get mad at me. She just tried to help me in any way that she could. She had a pretty good knack of knowing when to ask me if I needed help, when just to standby, and I guess, pray for me. It was probably tougher on my wife, because she would see me just curled up in a ball, because I was in a lot of pain and there was really nothing she could do. She'd try to adjust things and I probably snapped at her a number of times. Care-givers really need to be strong and to be able to take some negativity or verbal abuse, such as "That isn't going to work; I don't need that."

I'm just having a hard time with my kids. It seems like they don't want to hear it, but I feel that if they can really know how I feel, that it would make them more comfortable. I know my kids felt helpless, that they couldn't do anything. So what I'm going to do is probably write a letter to my boys—really tell them how I feel and hopefully it will make them more comfortable.

Some people sort of seemed to be afraid of getting together. I guess I'm sort of the same way. I mean they didn't know what I was going through. I don't think that they really wanted to know. Some of my musician friends were just really uncomfortable going to the hospital. But yet, as soon as they started playing music, it changed. It was like they were in a different place.

Sexual Life

(The day my prostate was removed) I didn't function sexually anymore. I don't think it's going to be a really big issue because sex hadn't been a big part of our life prior to the surgery.

Communication with Others

I think that sometimes it's just really hard for people to know how to talk to patients. But, once you start talking to people, then they become more comfortable—almost instantly. I've gone through periods of time where I was having bad days and we were living with my mother-in-law. She had friends over and they would tell me how good I looked. I said, "Please don't say that because I know that I don't look good. I feel horrible."

A lot of people tell me I'm really courageous. I don't feel like I'm courageous. I think that it's the people that had to live with me and deal with things, like my wife being a caregiver and then also my kids. Those are the people that are courageous to stay with a patient and give them what they need and basically not freak out.

Social Life

My social life was almost zero. But my social life wasn't important to me. I didn't feel I was missing out on things. Most of the time, I felt so bad that I didn't worry about socializing.

Non-Cancer Medical Problems and Stresses

About halfway through the chemo, I ended up with a bleeding ulcer. It made life really miserable. But the doctor figured out what it was and I just got off the medication that they were giving me. That issue is basically in my past now.

We were struggling with our finances. My wife was struggling with some pain. She had a hip replacement, and her other hip that wasn't operated on was starting to bother her more and more. This became a real issue last year in my recovery because it had gotten so bad she ended up in a wheelchair for a couple of months waiting for the surgery. My granddaughter was born with major brain damage. In the middle of chemo, my mother-in-law was having issues. We had to move into her house to help her out. We ended up throwing out 75% of our possessions just because I didn't want to pay for storage.

Coping with Having Cancer

After surgery, I was in no pain and no discomfort. I was on a morphine drip. Fifteen hours after surgery I was on my phone, texting my craftsmen and sending out emails to clients. Work has really helped me. I think a lot of things came to a halt through the cancer treatments. But I feel very fortunate that I do architectural design work, so a lot of my work is just sitting behind a desk. Actually doing design work has really helped me cope through some of the side effects of the chemo. It sort of took my mind off of what I was going through. There were other times where it didn't do much to help me. *(However),* what would help is finding something that keeps your mind off discomfort. After my surgery, I'd always be listening to music. Music would be on while I was going through all my procedures when I was in the hospital. It really seemed to help me a lot. I tend to latch onto lyrics that apply to my life. One of my favorites is by Jesse Winchester: "All That We Have Is Now."

(Another) thing that I seem to be attracted to is music about God, and especially about strength through God. I prayed for strength in getting through all the procedures. My wife also really helped with that. Every time I'd have a procedure, I would be able to say a little prayer to give me strength to get through this and see another day.

I didn't know if it was saying the prayer, or if it was the fact that my wife was always with me and always called. I don't think she's calm on the inside, but her calmness on the outside I think really helped me get through everything, without just freaking out and worrying about stuff and being negative.

I watched TV shows where they would fix up cars, *Family Feud* (*TV game show*) and John Wayne movies. I normally wouldn't watch these—sometimes you just have to space out on stupid things. One thing that helped me a lot was our little dog. He was always around, always by my side. When I was in my sick room, and after surgery, he'd come and then take sunbaths with me. Pets can be really therapeutic. We had two cats. They would come in and visit with me if the dog was out of the house. These things helped me cope to deal with the pain and all the issues that come along with cancer.

Satisfaction with Medical Care During Treatment

I felt really comfortable with (*my oncologist*). The department was good. I feel that it isn't one doctor, that it's a team. The doctors share all of their information with the other doctors, so when I go to another doctor, they pull up my files—they see everything that the other doctors have done. They have a lot of nurses that would help me deal with any sort of issues that I had. When I was going through chemo, they prescribed a couple of anti-nausea medications. On my second round of chemo, I was getting nauseated. (*The nurse then said*): "You're taking both of your medications, aren't you?" I said, "No, I have only taken one," to which the nurse replied, "You're supposed to (*also*) be taking this other one." By the time I got back home, I got a call from the pharmacy saying that the prescription had been filled. They were really on the spot in taking care of everything. My surgeons and oncologist were concerned about any depression and anxiety that I might have and offered help, which I felt I didn't need. I really had a deep trust in what the doctors and physicians said— that they would do something to make me more comfortable.

LON: *Colon Cancer, Stage III, 70 years old, male, disease-free two years*

Life One Year Before Diagnosis

I felt hopeless, utterly hopeless. I have late stage Type 2 diabetes, so both legs have swelled up to almost elephantiasis size. Then I started getting sores and lesions on my right ankle and they really swelled up—became painful. I was taking zinc oxide, some antibiotics, and anti-swelling medications. It feels good now, but it was so painful before. Since I didn't have a car I had to walk everywhere. I also have a degenerative disc disease *(congenital back defect)*, which effects my lower and upper back. So when I'm walking and if I have a backpack on, I'll start getting charley horse in my upper back and I have to stop and rest and take a breath about every two blocks. It becomes extremely painful. I also have AFib *(atrial fibrillation of the heart)*, which is an irregular heartbeat. These three medical problems that I had for some time before my having colon cancer added to my emotional instability and generally depressed, gloomy outlook. I simply wanted to be left alone and die.

Diagnosis of Colorectal Cancer

I had been feeling extremely listless and very depressed. I knew something was terribly wrong. It was a progressively deteriorating situation, affecting the rest of my body. I isolated myself almost entirely. But I figured I could take care of myself—find the strength necessary to fight whatever was attacking me. My doctor said, "You're going in for a colonoscopy." They found this mass about the size of a man's fist.

Treatment and Treatment Side Effects

I went in for surgery, and there was the mass, almost three times the size they thought it was. The cancer went down three inches into my lower colon, so the surgeon had to remove that, of course. Then they tied it back up so I don't have a colostomy bag. They also found 27 to 29 lymph nodes that were cancerous. The surgeon said that I had a 7% chance of successful recovery. They had me so anesthetized I really didn't feel any pain until probably day three when it became extremely painful. On a numbered scale of zero to 10 *(10 was the highest degree of pain)*, it was well beyond number 10.

I had chemo every other week for six months. I had diarrhea, constipation, hot sweats, and sores all over my body, worse than shingles, joints aching all the time, teeth hurting, gums bleeding, tremendous headaches. I was falling down all the time, so I had to learn how to walk again. Just the thought of food made me nauseous for about the first month. The doctor and I had an extremely good relationship. I said to him, "I can't do this anymore." He said, "We'll give it two more months." I was in so much pain, and it wasn't just the pain, it was mental chaos.

Quality of Life During Treatment

Emotional State

I just withdrew within myself and tried to call on some type of inner strength.

Relationships with Family, Friends, and Acquaintances

My wife went through this entire thing with me. She had to go through six months of living hell. I'm sure that I was just a terrible person she had to deal with because I was in constant pain. It ended up with us getting a divorce because of the stress. In addition to my wife, my wife's best friend, strangers that my wife knew, and volleyball teammates came forth at my lowest point halfway through chemo. They saved the day, along with Toby, our dog.

I have two sons. One is very supportive. He's a good guy, a good kid, and just a joy. He sends me gifts for my birthday and cards. He came a couple of times to visit, but he lives all over the place. It's difficult for him to stop what he's doing and take time off. My second son was always a difficult child and has been in trouble since he got divorced. I have a love-hate relationship with him.

Coping with Having Cancer

A lot of times when I was recovering *(I was)* trying to become "normal" again. I always saw it as you play the cards you're dealt. You would rather not have cancer, and not have AFib, but you've got it. There's no sense complaining.

Pets

Our dog Toby, who also saved the day, would jump up on my bed every single morning. He would snuggle with me for about five, 10 minutes. If I were feeling poorly and was not going to be getting up that day, he would come and lie down by the side of the bed and I would pet him. Every single morning Toby was there.

Satisfaction with Medical Care During Treatment

If you're going to get cancer, go to *(my medical center)*. They literally saved my life. There's no question about it. The surgeon did an excellent job, a super job, along with my medical oncologist, with whom I unburdened all my hopes and fears. I don't know how I got my oncologist as my doctor, but thank God. I would not be here without him. The doctor who did the colonoscopy and the nurses were just fabulous, especially at the cancer center. Very, very supportive and very, very kind and gentle.

CAROL R.: *Colon Cancer, Stage III, 78 years old, female, disease-free 3.5 years*

Life One Year Before Diagnosis

We just had a pretty normal life. I was very healthy. We were just very busy people. Although we live in a farm, we don't actually farm anymore. We have a lot of acreage to take care of and we have rental property also. So, it just seems like we're always doing something and it was usually manual labor—hard work. There was a certain amount of pressure, but not bad pressure. We also had a lot of pleasure. We traveled a lot and we had enjoyed 18 years of retirement. I felt good. I never worried about being sick. I never really thought about ever having anything serious. I never went to a doctor and I didn't have a colonoscopy. I just didn't think I needed it.

Diagnosis of Colorectal Cancer

This thing in my stomach started hurting and it progressively got to be more painful. It wasn't too long before I actually decided I better go to the emergency room. The doctor did a lot of tests and then he called me. He said it was a growth. (*That I had colon cancer*) didn't hit me hard. I just never felt shocked. I don't think I was worried at all. I don't know if it's a Midwestern thing or if it's the way I was raised, you just deal with what you have to deal with. You plow through it as much as you can. All I wanted to do is get on with it, get it done, and get my life back.

Treatment and Treatment Side Effects

The surgery was done a few days after the emergency room. The surgeon confirmed it was cancer. I think they took out everything they could, like the appendix, anywhere where the cancer could spread. It was the easiest surgery I ever had. I recovered really well from that.

It took four weeks before I started with chemo. The doctor told me that I would have chemo for at least eight treatments, but "we're going for the 12 treatments. We're going for a cure. We're not going for anything else but a cure." That jacked me right up.

I had very, very little pain. However, chemo took a lot out of me. It really zapped me. Maybe three to four days after the chemo treatment, in the beginning, it didn't bother me too much. It got worse, and towards the last two to three treatments, I had no good days between treatments. It was just like a horrible flu. I threw up once or twice, had diarrhea and weakness. I had fatigue at the beginning of chemo through several years later, and I still don't have my stamina back. I just generally felt lousy. Peripheral neuropathy started maybe three quarters of the way through the chemo. It progressively got worse. I kind of conditioned myself that it probably wasn't going to go away, but that's a small price to pay. I ended up having permanent neuropathy in my legs, feet, hands, and fingers. I lost my balance a lot because of my feet, and my legs were so numb a lot of the time, and it was hard to walk normally. I would not have been able to handle having chemo if I hadn't been in such good shape. I was strong and basically healthy *(before having had colon cancer)*.

Quality of Life During Treatment

Emotional State

I didn't want to be around sad people or complaining people or depressed people. I didn't want to be pulled down.

Relationships with Family, Friends, and Acquaintances

My husband was there every second and very, very supportive. My kids were very supportive. I don't know what I would have done *(without that)*. I did have a lot of support from friends too. People came out of the woodwork who I didn't even expect would know

I have anything wrong with me, but I guess word travels a little. I had the ideal situation I'd say of having support, right there with me. I just strongly feel that was why I recovered so quickly. My heart goes out to people that don't have that. I don't know how people do this alone.

Coping with Having Cancer

I did what I had to do, that was it. I had to keep my mind in the right place. I couldn't let myself think of anything else except making this all better. I never thought I'd die. There was so little I could do to help myself. I lost control of my bowels, my urination, my appetite, my active life, the work that I knew was sitting out there that I should have been doing. I looked for things to be in control of and that probably helped me in my recovery. Whether I was nauseous or not, I ate. That gave me a little empowerment. I never complained, or tried to never complain about having cancer. That's another thing where I thought I could have control. Maybe I sought control because I lost so much control and you're so dependent on everybody. That's not the way I've been all my life.

Religion

I also looked at spirituality in a different way. I know that I felt God. Why was He helping me? I haven't been a very nice person during my life. *(There was just unbelievable peace)* whenever I had to do something that I was uneasy about. I know that was God.

Satisfaction with Medical Care During Treatment

I can't believe such good people exist. They're like unearthly. There's so much information in my oncologist's mind that I just don't know how he holds it all. Another asset, and probably right up alongside my family, were the chemo nurses. They were unbelievable. People are really sick from chemo. The nurses were unbelievably compassionate, gentle and just caring. I just don't know they can give so much of themselves. I feel I had the best care I could possibly get.

IRENE M.: *Colon Cancer, Stage III, 80 years old, female, disease-free three years*

Life One Year Before Diagnosis

My husband had passed away *(two years before I was diagnosed with colon cancer.)* I was his caregiver for five years. He had a coronary, many strokes, and Alzheimer's. He got very nasty at the end. Sometimes he took his cane and battered me with it. I had to keep reminding myself that that wasn't him, it was the disease. Towards the end, emotionally and physically, there was just nothing left of me. Then *(after his death)* there was dealing with all the other things, like his name on all the bills. I've had chronic upper respiratory problems since I was five or six years old, coronary artery disease when 70 years old, chronic kidney disease, Stage III, and the biggest is the non-alcoholic liver disease (NASH) when *(I was)* 68 years old.

Diagnosis of Colorectal Cancer

It wasn't a normal going to the bathroom. It would be every 15 minutes—I would get the urge and nothing was there. Or, I would have a lot of bloating and gas. I went to my primary care doctor and he felt I was eating too many salads. I asked him did he think I should have a colonoscopy, and he thought I didn't need one until I was 80 *(was 78 years old at that time)*. My family said, "Mom, go get a colonoscopy." So, I did that and I had colon cancer, Stage III. I just froze. Fortunately I had a family member with me.

Treatment and Treatment Side Effects

I was operated on using a laparoscope and *(part of my colon was removed)*. The recovery was faster than I had anticipated. The first four days *(after the surgery)* I slept on a reclining chair that had an electric button, so when I wanted to get up all I had to do was push the button and it almost had me in a standing position. It was less painful because you're pulling a muscle when you lie flat. *(After that)* I was able to manage lying in bed and during the day I tried to do little things. The first three weeks I had to have help in the house. Then I started to go for walks. It might have been six weeks that I couldn't drive. I don't think I felt frustrated *(while I was recovering)*. I just thought it was part of the healing process.

Quality of Life During Treatment

Relationship with Family, Friends, and Acquaintances

I am blessed with four wonderful children. They were all there. They were very supportive. I think they were very frightened. My daughter-in-law and my daughter took turns staying overnight with me at the hospital. These poor girls slept on a chair and my daughter took a couple of days off so they took turns, making sure that I had something to eat. *(In the six weeks after surgery when I couldn't drive)*, my family was there making sure I got to wherever I had to go. I also made a list of things I needed, so when they came I could just hand the list to them. I have great neighbors. Somebody would call and say, "I'm going to CVS *(pharmacy)*." I'd say, "Could you pick up my medicine?"

Satisfaction with Medical Care During Treatment

(My medical care from my surgeon and his team) was wonderful. I couldn't ask for a better team. *(However)* three days before my

operation I went to my primary care doctor and he said, "You don't need robotics *(laparoscopy)*. They'll only charge you $8,000 more." That was when I froze. I expected some support from him and it wasn't there. I think I was more crushed by that whole thing than I was about the operation and having cancer, because this *(doctor and his wife)* were my friends.

KAYW: *Colon Cancer, Stage I, 82 years old, female, disease-free three years (KAYW is disabled; interview was conducted with her husband)*

Life One Year Before Diagnosis

My wife was very, very weak. She was diagnosed as anemic and had to have blood infusions about every three months. This went on for a year. That year it really kept down her ability to function. We decided to just wait and see. Prior to having anemia, KayW had a major stroke and heart problems. Further, two of our sons had died. One was killed in a work accident when he was 38 years old. The oldest son was 58 years old and died of a heart attack two years ago. That was very, very difficult.

Diagnosis of Colorectal Cancer

After a year, the doctor said KayW should go to a gynecologist and get checked out. An ultrasound was conducted in 2015 and she had a tumor the size of a small orange. It didn't really shake her up that much to be diagnosed with having colon cancer. She didn't get depressed except maybe a few times or just for a few minutes. It was like, "Let's go do something about it." It seemed as though it really didn't affect her that much because she had been through having heart problems and a major stroke in 2008. Maybe in her mind she just thought, "Oh, here comes another one."

Treatment and Treatment Side Effects

As KayW only had Stage I colon cancer, she only needed surgery. We did get a good surgeon and he did the surgery laparoscopically. Twenty-five percent of her colon was taken out. She came home in about two days. Then maybe in a week she was doing fine. The only thing we're doing now is for my wife to have follow-up blood tests.

Quality of Life During Treatment

Non-Cancer Medical Problems

She wasn't diagnosed with having Alzheimer's until 2016, when it really started affecting her. Right now, she's probably in late stage— Stage IV *(highest is Stage V)*. I had to do a lot more for her in 2016. I help her bathe, get her dressed, and put her pajamas on. It is the Lord that's provided me with the ability to go out to sort, clean, and do the wash to take care of her. We've just been doing it together up until now. We haven't really had to hire anybody.

Coping with Having Cancer

You can't explain the number of people who prayed for KayW. That's just a tremendous benefit. Even when we go to church, they are all coming up to her. They all love her. If I think I need something, they'll come right over. I haven't gotten to that point yet *(of needing to do that)*, but it may happen in the future.

Satisfaction with Medical Care During Treatment

The medical care was excellent. We didn't have any problems with the doctors and nurses or anything. Even with the tumor that large, the surgeon was pretty upbeat. "We'll go in, and get it out of there."

MYRNA: *Colon Cancer, Stage II, 82 years old, female, disease-free 1.5 years*

Life One Year Before Diagnosis

One year before my diagnosis things were not good with me. My spouse had died in June 2015 when we were in Europe *(two years before my diagnosis with cancer)*. It was a traumatic experience. Half of me died when my spouse died. With her death, it was difficult to do things with friends, and in particular, couples. However, physically I was feeling great. I had no obvious symptoms. I didn't have much of a clue about what was going on somatically *(with my body)*. My relationships with family were great. I have a daughter and son-in-law, and several nieces and nephews, and we stay in touch. But, all my sisters have died, the last one being two years ago. I have friends and a support system. I was at the gym every day and was still seeing patients as a volunteer *(I'm a psychologist)*.

Diagnosis of Colorectal Cancer

I was experiencing some dyspnea and shortness of breath and I couldn't understand why I was having these things. There were no other symptoms. I kept delaying and delaying. I decided that I would go and see my internist. He did some blood work and, lo and behold, my internist called and said, "Get yourself to the hospital. Your hemoglobin is high (6.1.)," which indicates that I'm bleeding someplace. A colonoscopy was done and sure enough, it was Stage II colon cancer.

Treatment and Treatment Side Effects

I was given four options as to what to do: (1) radical surgery, but since it was on the right side, it would mean that I wouldn't have to have an ostomy bag, which was good, (2) radiation *or* chemo, or (3) a combination of radiation and chemo. The fourth option was doing nothing. If I did nothing, I had three to six months to live. I chose the radical surgery because I didn't want to put myself through chemo and radiation. A third of the right side of my colon was removed, as well as the cecum *(pouch connecting small and large intestines)* and appendix. Also, 46 lymph nodes were removed. Before the surgery I wanted to know what kind of support I was going to be getting because I knew that I was going to be needing emotional support and it was all explained to me.

Quality of Life During Treatment

Emotional State

It was kind of scary stuff. But I steeled myself to cancer possibly occurring elsewhere, dying, and living uncomfortably. I was sad and a bit frightened about going through the recovery alone. I just hunkered down. I didn't go out. My emotional state was a state of both gratitude for a successful surgery and anxiety about what lay ahead for me at my advanced age.

Relationships with Family, Friends, and Acquaintances

My daughter was a godsend. She checked in with me by phone or text daily, from when I was diagnosed through the present. When I was discharged from the hospital, my daughter was with me for a week after that.

Coping During Treatment

While in the hospital I watched a lot of Netflix *(movies, TV shows)*. I read stuff voraciously.

Satisfaction with Medical Care During Treatment

I had a very, very good surgeon. She was just marvelous. The surgeon and all of the residents and fellows that were with the surgeon were very eager to understand my situation. The ability of the oncology fellow to listen to *better understand* rather than *respond* was extraordinary. Then the surgeon and all of the residents and fellows who were with the surgeon were very eager to understand my situation. You could see the learning in their eyes. They were just wonderful. I couldn't have asked for anything better.

However, two mistakes had almost been made, but I caught them. The first mistake had to do with being given a blood thinner. I said, "I don't think I should have this because my hemoglobin was 6.1 when I came into the hospital." I thought that my hemoglobin level was not creeping up yet and a blood thinner was only going to make it worse. My oncologist agreed with me. The next mistake was when I needed to be transfused again, the nurse came in with the blood in a bag, labeled A– *(negative)*. I said "Stop—I'm A+ *(positive)*." Other than that I really have no complaints. I think that there are systemic issues everywhere. But I also think that we patients really need to be in charge, no matter how sick we are. The mistakes were all well-meaning, but there are slips.

KATHERINE W.: *Colon Cancer, disease stage not known, 86 years old, female, disease-free four years*

Life One Year Before Diagnosis

I was feeling great—no problems with my children or relatives. There were no medical problems or other stresses in my life.

Diagnosis of Colorectal Cancer

I started having some stomach cramps. I had no bleeding, nothing unusual. But it just got worse. I got through Christmas and I said, "We've got to do something." I went to a gastroenterologist and he said, "I should have done a colonoscopy on you. But you were already 80 years old—I didn't think it was necessary." Then he did a colonoscopy and he came out and said, "I'm sorry to tell you, but

I swear that it's colon cancer." My gastroenterologist was so upset and so apologetic. I'm a pretty calm person and I wasn't extremely upset. Of course, I didn't like it. I just said, "Well, let's get through it." I did have a lot of faith. I did talk to my minister and he gave me lots of good advice. I just knew that I would get through it and do what I had to do.

I told my children right away. They were very concerned. They said, "We'll get through it." That's kind of how we accept everything. We've had some other things in our lives and we just got through it. I have a wonderful support group of friends and they were concerned. They just said, "Let us know what we can do." Most of my friends are from the church, but not all of them.

Treatment and Treatment Side Effects

I had surgery. The right side of my colon was removed. They got all the cancer out. I had no bags *(colostomy)*. I had no further treatment. I had no more pain than what you might have after surgery. It was laparoscopic. It was mild compared to what I could have had. Two weeks after I had surgery I was told that I did not have to have any chemo or anything. It was wonderful—I have a second life.

Quality of Life During Treatment

Functioning

After two weeks I was doing whatever I wanted to do. I got over it very quickly.

Relationships with Family, Friends, and Acquaintances

My son came in and stayed with me. He was my helper. He made me get up, walk, drink. You had to do everything he said. He was a slave driver.

My friends from the church came to visit, and it's not only my friends from church, but other friends of mine who were very supportive.

Coping with Having Cancer

I think my attitude *(helped me cope)*. I'm a very independent person. Also, I have a son in town and he was involved—he checked up on me. I didn't need anything *(to help me cope)* that I did not get.

Satisfaction with Medical Care During Treatment

It was absolutely wonderful. I absolutely couldn't have asked for better care. I had a wonderful doctor. I could not recommend him enough. The nurses were excellent, just wonderful. I cried when I left one of them, telling her, "You've been so good to me." It was just an emotional thing because she was so good.

MARIE K.: *Colon Cancer, disease stage not known, 87 years old, female, disease-free five years*

Life One Year Before Diagnosis

I wasn't being held back from anything. I pretty much pushed forward to do anything. I am married and have three children. I have ups and downs with everybody, but nothing really serious—I mean it's just normal. We had friends when we lived in *(prior city)*. We did a lot together. Since we moved to where we are now, I didn't have as many friends as I had. There are a few, but now I'm getting older. My friends are dying, unfortunately.

Diagnosis of Colorectal Cancer

I have irritable bowel syndrome. I've had it since I was in my 20s. To me, life is full of stress, so it affects the stomach. That's the way I've been for many years. I just probably got to the point that I've got to find out and make sure everything is OK. I just thought I should have another colonoscopy. I finally went to a gastroenterologist. I ended up having a colonoscopy and he's the one that found the cancer.

Treatment and Treatment Side Effects

I was so busy that month getting ready for surgery because I had to go for tests to make sure everything was in order. You go for one test and for another test. I didn't have time to sit down and worry about it. I was upset of course. I was just trying to get through this, one step at a time. The surgeon took out quite a bit of the colon *(done laparoscopically)*. It was a breeze. I felt so good afterwards. I wasn't in any pain. There was no external bag *(colostomy)*. I didn't have to have chemo at all. It took about a month to recover. I was rarely restricted on anything because the surgery I had was so minor. I just did really well. However, even several months *(after the surgery),* you'll have your days where you're a little bit slower, and you take it easy. That's what I did. Actually, it wasn't bad at all.

Quality of Life During Treatment

Emotional State

My husband was very supportive, helped me big time. But there are times you do have to rely on yourself. I find if I can't handle the whole thing, I say, "OK, what's the next step?" That's the way I've had to do it and that is something you have to acquire. I couldn't go to pieces.

Relationships with Family, Friends, and Acquaintances.

We pretty much could handle *(my having surgery)* ourselves. Everybody sort of helped out here and there. Our youngest son did an awful lot for us during that time. The rest of the children came in and did what they could. We did very well because of that. We definitely had friends who helped. A cardiac nurse lives down the street. She had offered to help if we needed her, which we did, of course. Another neighbor, who lived just across the street, shoveled the snow and sent over things. I'm panicking now because we don't have those people, one died and the other one moved. We have a few *(neighbors)* here that I or my husband could call upon.

Other Non-Cancer Medical Problems and Stressful Events

My biggest stress is when my son died. He had lung cancer. It was too far advanced to do anything.

Coping with Having Cancer During Treatment

Our minister was very active at the church and I saw him. However, everything went pretty well, really. I was lucky, very lucky.

Satisfaction with Medical Care During Treatment

I really did feel that I got good medical care. The surgeon and nurses were excellent. The surgeon answered every question as best as he could.

AFTER TREATMENT AND THROUGH SURVIVORSHIP

JIM M.: *Colorectal Cancer, Stage IV, 68 years old, male, disease-free one year*

Long-Term Treatment Side Effects

Neuropathy has probably been the biggest ongoing side effect from the chemo. I still have neuropathy. *(The problem with)* my fingers and toes *(is)* making it hard to get back into running. I have a hard time walking; sometimes my balance is off. I can do my work—I can do a lot of things—but there's still some numbness in my fingers. I have a hard time turning pages sometimes, like newspapers or books.

Quality of Life after Treatment and Through Survivorship

Regaining and/or Changing One's Life

I feel like I've been reborn and that I have my life back. It's wonderful. I try not to think about *(the negative things)* at all. I don't worry about cancer coming back. If it does, I'll deal with it at that time. I've told my wife that life's too short to worry, and if we worry, we won't enjoy our life.

One thing that I think is important is that I found that there are some things that I've lost going through everything, and some things have come back. But, "If I can't do something, then find something else to do." Running was a big part of my life. One of my big things in the recovery was to try to get back my strength through exercise. When the cancer hit, there was no exercising; you need to save your strength for fighting the disease. Occupational therapy lasted for six weeks and the physical therapy lasted for three months. I always looked forward to that. I wanted to get back in shape; the chemo left me so weak. The physical therapist asked me "What are your goals?" I said, "If you really want to know, I want to run a half marathon again." The physical therapist really worked hard on getting me back jogging—and I did. I hope that I'll be able to run again. It still is a struggle, but I feel that it's really an important part of recovery. But, in the meantime, I work out a lot on the elliptical machine, which is probably the closest thing that you can do exercise-wise to running. With the neuropathy in my fingers, I can't do all the things I want to do. *(In making a rabbit cage)*, I was working with my hands and it was nice to be able to do something again with my hands. I feel really blessed that I really enjoy my work. Work has been another therapy post-cancer.

Coping with Having Had Cancer

I enjoy talking to people about the journey that I've been through. One of the things that has helped me is talking with people and seeing how people are struggling with an issue and being able to help them a little bit. In talking with other people who had cancer, I get the feeling that <u>I'm not alone in this</u>. I try to latch onto the people that are positive—that they are trying to make life better for themselves.

Satisfaction with Medical Care after Treatment and Through Survivorship

The *(medical)* care going through it and then often post-chemo has just been top-rate. Other than wishing the team could have helped more in my dealing with neuropathy from the chemo, there haven't been any issues that I think "Why aren't they doing this or that for me?" It's always "they're doing so much more than what I really expected to get." What I hope that the medical profession can do for every patient is make them comfortable. I feel I've gotten that through all my experiences. They always try to make me comfortable. They are always concerned about me. I really love that about my doctors and the hospital. I can't think of anything that I would have needed that wasn't provided to me. The cancer center has a lot of resources: a good library and an infusion center with wonderful caring nurses. There were also nurses that were available that could help me with any issues (diet, medication, etc.). I feel that I had an excellent team that was concerned about my comfort and well-being.

Overall Impact of Having Had Cancer

Positive Effects

I don't regret having cancer because as I was going through everything, I felt that I was becoming stronger, not physically, but mentally, and I think emotionally too. "OK, I can deal with this." I don't feel like I lost a year of my life. I'm not fearful of cancer coming back. I feel like I have a new life. That's really a positive *(effect)* that I've gotten from going through *(having had cancer)*—seeing that I can get through it.

Life is probably better now for me than before I had cancer. It's triggered me to reorganize my business to where I really wanted it and can enjoy it more. I just feel that I'm a lot more comfortable with myself than I was before cancer. I enjoy talking to people about the journey that I've been through. One of the things that has helped me is talking with people and seeing how people are struggling with an issue and being able to help them a little bit. In talking with other people who had cancer, I get the feeling that *I'm not alone in this.*

Advice

I *(met with)* an old high school friend who has a colostomy bag. I think that sharing experiences can really be good for cancer patients because then you don't feel alone. You feel like a lot of people are going through this, how they are dealing with it. Look for the positives and don't dwell on the negatives. Cancer is life-changing and you can lose a lot. There are things you can't change. You just have to look at the positives. When you do, I think it makes your life a lot more enjoyable. I really think that people, especially older people that are retired—have lost a big chunk in their life *(as a result of being retired)*. They really need, whether they have cancer or not, to find something that they're passionate about.

LON, *Colon Cancer, Stage III, 70 years old, male, disease-free two years*

Long-Term Treatment Side Effects

I still have issues like balance. My short-term memory was wiped out because of the chemo drugs. I had to force myself, in my mind, to take insignificant tasks and break them down into a step-by-step flow chart. That's the only way I could cope with that.

Quality of Life after Treatment Through Survivorship

Emotional State

I'm a fighter, a very competitive person. I felt "this too shall pass." What doesn't kill me makes me stronger. It is as if I had to have cancer to really come alive. I needed such a dramatic shock in my life to get me out of the doldrums, to at least help with the physical problems that I had. If I hadn't had cancer, I would have continued on that path and would probably be dead by now.

Relationships with Family, Friends, and Acquaintances

I think seeing the face of death and the possibility that you are seeing someone die in front of you is very frightening for people. I consider the people in our group at Gilda's Club (*provides services for cancer patients*) more as friends than anybody that I know. When you've been consumed by a nightmare, you really want to spend a lot of time with other people who have gone through a similar experience. Those are the ones you think who will understand and care.

Regaining and/or Changing One's Life

(*Since childhood*), people have always told me that I can't do it, that I'm too small, I'm too slow. That has always been the impetus and igniter for me to say, "Yes, I will." (*However, at first, when I had been diagnosed as having colon cancer and treated*), I had isolated myself. It was a foolish, foolish thing to do. You have to have an indomitable will and overpowering belief in yourself. I'm a great believer in the old Greek idea of mind, body, and spirit together. That's the reason why I started working out almost two years ago, in order to get my body back to the point where I could do things. I had strength because my mind was returning, but it was so very, very slow. I'm not anywhere near where I'd like to be. It's *(been)* going on for three years now. I thought it was going to take just six months. The "new me," the "I can" me, is like 75%–80% "I can," and maybe not even 15%–20% "I can't." On the "I can" days, I just keep on thinking positive thoughts. "I can do this." My body is sound again. My mind is recovering. The frustration comes because I can't do the things I used to do with ease. I have to do them over and over again, and I have to be patient. Volleyball was my life, basketball too, and riding my bike. We used to go to volleyball tournaments virtually every weekend during the winter. But I can't play basketball or volleyball, and I can't ride my bike right now. It scares me because of my imbalance. I miss that so much. At some point, though, I'm going to be able to ride my bicycle again. I do a lot of reading. I love to read and I just lose myself in books. I've played chess for maybe 25 years. When I play chess, I can completely remove myself from any atmosphere in which I'm involved. I take the Relaxation Guided Imagery class (RGI) in Gilda's Club *(an organization designed to help cancer patients)*. Our mentor takes us traveling within our minds to a safe place through guided imagery. And then you give yourself positive feedback: "Your body is strong; it can recover. Your mind is strong." Without that, without working out, I probably would have done something dangerous to myself.

Now I have fun and am enjoying life to the fullest. I go out; I do what I want to do. I'm living by myself. I am my own master. I've got new friends now. My body is feeling better than it has been in the last 30 years. My mind is recovering. I would like to have companionship, but I'm not willing to give up certain parts of my personal life, such as going to the library and doing my research. I'm writing a novel, a short story, and I'm trying to write a play. I'm just doing the things that I've really wanted to do all along. *(In the past)*, there was always something else that I was supposed to be doing.

Coping with Having Had Cancer

What helped me cope was joining Gilda's Club. Everybody knows everybody and it's just a very positive thing. Generally speaking, when I'm in trouble, I withdraw into myself. But I choose to communicate with other people in this very warm, comforting, and inclusive group who have cancer, because we know something other people don't. I'm going to become what's called an Ambassador for Gilda's Club. We go to small civic groups, like the PTA *(Parent-Teacher Association)*. I explained to them what my situation was and how I overcame it and what I went through when I had chemo. It feels good to share this with other people because I think it's a message of hope. I want to help others to see that a fulfilling life is possible after the potential death sentence of cancer, if you work hard, gain confidence, and never, never give up. In addition, I have been transitioning to Buddhism for about three to four years. The Buddhist religion aligns much more with my thoughts of an afterlife, of a great spirit. One of the things that actually helped me was the concept of "We are all one." It fit right into where I was going.

Overall Impact of Having Had Cancer

Negative and Positive Effects

Probably the biggest negative thing is accepting the fact that there are certain things I'll never do again. I'll never play basketball again. I'll never play volleyball again.

Advice

I would say the worst thing you can do when you're diagnosed with cancer is to isolate yourself. At that moment, you have got to reach out. There's a whole bunch of people and a whole bunch of organizations that are there to help you through this thing. But you have got to reach out to other people. You cannot do this by yourself. I would strongly recommend contacting organizations like Gilda's Club and having at least weekly meetings with others in the same situation. It's amazing the bonds you form. When recovering from cancer, you need to have at least one very positive point in your life. Hopefully you have many, but you need to get one because it's kind of an anchor that you have to hang onto if the "I can't" rises up and says, "No, I can't." You need that point of light.

CAROL R.: *Colon Cancer, Stage III, 78 years old, female, disease-free 3.5 years*

Quality of Life after Treatment and Through Survivorship

Emotional State

One thing that probably has bothered me is whenever I get a twinge or a stomachache, I think, "It's starting again." I asked the doctor, "When do you stop thinking that way?" He said. "Most people never do. It just seems to be a normal reaction."

Regaining and/or Changing One's Life

I guess I had the ideal cancer situation: good support and such good people helping me to get better. I can't think of anything that I would have needed that I didn't have. However, it took me three years to get back to feeling normal. I did what I could to make myself healthy again and just not dwell on sadness. My lifestyle has changed. I don't know if it's changed because of the cancer, but it's probably also changed because I'm getting older and slowing down, although I think cancer did me in. I just don't have the stamina anymore to do things, and chemo caused balance and other neuropathy problems that don't allow me to do things I used to like to do. I don't feel we can travel anymore—we loved to do that. My husband and I used to hike. Now, we stroll, and not very far. I keep thinking, "I'm going to get that *(being active)* back," but I don't think I'm going to live long enough to get it back. I would like to be able to still do some of the things we used to do. I like to refinish furniture. I've always done that, but not during our retirement so much. But now, I'm getting back into that a little bit and I enjoy that. I love to read. I spend a lot of time reading, day in, day out. I'd like to be more physically active, but it just takes time. I'm not there yet—maybe next year. I certainly feel a lot better now than I did a year ago or a year before that. I'd say I'm doing pretty good, but I always like to be better.

Prior Experiences That Helped with Coping

When you have difficult situations, like my having a tough, disciplinarian father and a loving but stern mother, you get a muscle hardened to get through it. I think nobody lives a number of years without having difficulties and I think that strengthens you for the really hard things coming up.

Overall Impact of Having Had Cancer

Positive Effects

Maybe I've improved my life because of it. I think I'm a lot more compassionate, especially towards cancer people and kids a lot more. Little kids that get cancer look so sick. I wonder how they deal with it. I wonder how their parents deal with it. It's got to be so hard. I think *(having had cancer)* made me appreciate people more, made me appreciate the intelligence and absolute skill of the surgeons, doctors, and nurses. It's awesome. I never felt this way before. *(Having had cancer)* helped me a lot to see the goodness in people. I think it also strengthened my faith. I've seen a lot of strength in myself that I didn't know I had. I'm seeing some great things in my family that

I didn't know existed. I think I'd like to maybe be a volunteer, but not right now. I've got to probably get better myself.

Greatest Concerns

(One of my greatest concerns was) that my kids might get it. Another thing that kept me going was I want to be the survivor in our marriage. I want to help my husband go through the last of his life. I've got to be here for him. I just don't want him to have to suffer. That was a good thing to really realize that.

Advice

You can control your mind and see how you want to go through life. I think that the most important thing for me to do was to keep my mind in the right spot, not give into self-pity, or anger, or regret. You have to be brave as you possibly can.

Look at the person next to you in the chemo chairs—see how they're so sick. In my first chemo treatment, an old lady was right in the chair next to me. She looked at me and said, "This is your first time, I know. It's not so bad." That helped me feel pretty good. Do that to somebody else next to you in the next chemo chair.

IRENE M.: *Colon Cancer, Stage III, 80 years old, female, disease-free three years*

Quality of Life after Treatment and Through Survivorship

Emotional State

(Cancer) is always in my face. Now I go *(for follow-up medical appointments)* every six months. The anticipation is you get the blood work, you go for the CAT scan with the contrast and then you have to wait. You're waiting for that and you keep saying to your-

self, "It's going to be fine. There's nothing there. You're fine." You keep talking to yourself but there's that little voice inside you: "But, what if?" It's like someone I can't throw out of the house and say, "Go." So, it's always there. Then if you get an ache or a pain, it's like, "What was that?"

Non-Cancer Medical Problems

I don't allow my medical issues, chronic upper respiratory problems, coronary artery disease, chronic kidney disease, and my non-alcoholic liver disease interfere with my physical or emotional well-being. I'm able to be independent and do all the functions of daily living.

Coping with Having Had Cancer

I try to stay positive. I try to be active as I can. I give myself the 30 seconds of feeling sorry for myself, and then I go, "OK, you did your 30 seconds, now move on."

Religion, especially spirituality, is extremely important *(in coping with having had cancer)*. I prayed a lot. I go to Mass every Sunday. When I get up in the morning, before I put my feet on the floor, I thank God for another beautiful day, and that I hope that I make the most of this beautiful day. I do meditation. At night I go to bed with this very soft music and I say the rosary over and over again and I fall asleep.

Although I was a non-crafty person, *(by being a member of Gilda's Club—a support program for cancer patients)* I made jewelry. They're doing some kind of artwork with glass, so I think I'm going to try that. I do a lot of volunteer stuff. I open up the museum for a couple of hours. At the business school they have story hours, so I go up and read once a week to the little ones. You have no idea how much joy they give you. And then there is babysitting two great grandsons. Whenever Gilda's Club needs somebody, I just tell them, "Wherever you need me, put me." It doesn't matter what I do.

Coping Needs That Went Unmet

Everything seems to be available for every other types of cancer, which is good. But little is done for colon cancer, even having support groups.

The Impact of Prior Life Experiences on Coping

I was sexually abused by my stepfather when I was eight years old, and nobody believed me. It's shame-based—I didn't talk about it with anyone. I don't think you ever recover. I had a meltdown in my 40s related to the sexual abuse. We had a director at work who made overtures to me and I guess that triggered a lot of stuff. I was fortunate enough in getting a good therapist. But I guess overcoming it comes from God. You can knock me down, but I'm going to get up every time.

Satisfaction with Medical Care after Treatment and Survivorship

Between my primary care physician, my oncologist, and my gastroenterologist, my team has been excellent. I feel that they are concerned—wanting to keep on top of this—making sure I am 100% satisfied. They are wonderful.

Overall Impact of Having Had Cancer

Positive Effects

Cancer made me realize how fragile my life really is and each day is a blessing. I try to remember to do one act of kindness every single day, to try to be kind and forgiving.

Greatest Concerns

My greatest concern is that it will show up somewhere else, because I also know that cancer is very smart and it can show itself in a different form somewhere else in the body.

Advice

If you're not getting the kind of response from a doctor that you think you should be getting or at least exploring using some tests, like a simple colonoscopy, listen to your gut and get a second opinion. If my doctor had *(done a colonoscopy, my cancer)* would have been caught a lot earlier. No one knows your body better than you. Seek support. Don't do it alone—don't do it by yourself. Keep a sense of humor. I think my sense of humor gets me through life. Be positive. I guess I needed to be around people who say, "I'm five years cancer-free; I'm twelve years cancer-free; I'm twenty years cancer-free." That makes me smile. Yeah, people do beat this.

KAYW: *Colon Cancer, Stage I, 82 years old, female, disease-free three years (KAYW is disabled; interview was conducted with her husband)*

Long-Term Treatment Side Effects

With 25% of KayW's colon taken out, it affects her bowel movements. She can sometimes get a little constipated and then she'll get diarrhea.

Quality of Life after Treatment and Through Survivorship

Non-Cancer Medical Problems

She's at this point now *(in having Alzheimer's)* that it's hard for her to talk. She can visualize what she wants to say, but can't verbalize it. I was in the hospital and had a PICC line *(tube that goes into the arm and all the way up to a large vein near the heart),* and then I couldn't walk. I ended up deteriorating my right hip. I had a hip replacement and that's been great. But *(because of having the hip replacement),* I could see what was going to happen in the future—I had to keep my body strong. So, before the hip replacement, I got people to help *(with taking care of my wife)*, so that I could have the hip replacement done. They agreed to do it and it went fine. My son and daughter-in-law came over the night of the surgery and the next night. The night after that I was home. I just handled taking care of KayW after that.

Relationships with Family, Friends, and Acquaintances

Up until this point, the illnesses haven't really affected the relationships with the family or friends. Everybody's been really, really supportive. KayW and I do things together. Every morning I try to take her out to get breakfast some place. I think that helps her. We're Christians. We're believers and so that really helps. My kids and grandkids are just too busy to come over to our house, so we visit them. It's not because my wife has Alzheimer's that they don't come over. I remember back when we were younger, I didn't have a whole lot of interest in visiting my folks. However, when somebody needs something, we all pitch in and we do it for them. *(When asked about how drained he was about this)*: At times, maybe. Generally, it's been pretty good. Like last night she got up and I got up once and helped her. Fortunately she doesn't wander around really, because she gets right back to sleep. I'll lay there for a while and make sure she gets right back to sleep. That's not a problem.

Religion

We rely a lot on the Lord.

Overall Impact of Having Had Cancer

Greatest Concerns

KayW was concerned about what was going to happen after the surgery. The unknown is always a concern.

Advice

Do your own homework on doctors, treatments, diagnosis and everything. You really should do a lot of it yourself, get a full understanding of what's going on. Don't take one doctor's diagnosis. You're pretty much going to have to do this, and I think it's really daunting.

MYRNA: *Colon Cancer, Stage II, 82 years old, female, disease-free 1.5 years*

Quality of Life after Treatment and Through Survivorship

Emotional State

There's this thing that lurks in your body, and doesn't let you know that it's eating away at you until it gets to the point where it's so bad that getting rid of it is difficult. That's what's horrible about cancer and I think that's what's horrible about grief. I'm 82 years old and kind of have had a good life. I've been blessed. I'm more afraid of living than I am of dying. I wasn't interested in suffering and having my family suffer, and having to wind my way through the system without my spouse. However, while I don't feel horrible now about my wife's death, there is just an emptiness that doesn't go away. I wonder about recurrence or having other cancers, and have made plans to deal with that. While none of us can really know what we shall do until that occurs, I feel that heroics at this stage *(of my life)* are not something I would want for me or my family.

Regaining and/or Changing One's Life

Recuperation took about six months. I was grateful to be cleared to go back to daily exercise at the fitness center where I have been a member for scores of years. I continue to do exercises but have pared it down to five miles per day, instead of 10. Widowhood *(wife had died two years ago)* exacerbated problems in functioning *(due to hav-*

ing had cancer). With my spouse's death, I had to do a lot of things alone. I had great difficulty listening to and playing music. Seeing people for holidays was terribly difficult. I found great solace in being alone with my thoughts, feelings, and memories. I am much better now. I actually see more people, do more things, and practice the piano from time to time. I continue to see patients on a volunteer basis *(I'm a psychologist)* at the hospital, which is always very helpful for me. It always works when I can't get outside of myself. However, I don't think I'll get back to my life as it has been, largely due to my wife's death. But I'm getting back to *(some of my life now).* The nagging loss of my wife is constantly with me though.

Relationships with Family, Friends, and Acquaintances

Because my daughter calls or texts me daily, she was a great source of helping me cope, for which I am eternally grateful. She made a list of friends with whom I felt comfortable to do specific tasks with, like grocery shopping. I tapped my psychology buddies from the hospital. They were great at the supermarket. "Just tell me what you need" and off we would go. My daughter and son-in-law are both caring and loving as well as respecting distance and boundaries. They asked about my wishes and, as well, did not impose theirs. That's what made my daughter marvelous. That's what I mean by, "she left me alone." I feel blessed to have this family and a family of friends who do the same.

Other family members were and continue to be very supportive and respectful. I found that one couple, with whom my wife and I had been very, very close, came over. I could see how upset they were when they looked at me. I'm a rather well put-together person, and I must have looked horrible. I could see it on their faces, and I just didn't want to deal with them. Others would say, "You look great," when I looked horrible. I couldn't stand to see that reaction to me. I have made a conscious decision to *not* be with people who are kind of toxic for me—well meaning but saying things with that kind of look, "How sad you have cancer," and "Wow, you look great and keep up the good work." I don't care if people don't "get it," (under-stand what it is like to have cancer). I choose to be with people who are living their lives and letting me live mine, in spite of my cancer diagnosis. My friends who honor that are still good for me to be with. I am still *myself* and cancer did not change that.

Non-Cancer Medical Problems

I had hypothyroid problems, urinary tract infections, a reaction to antibiotics, and eczema (patches of rough, inflamed blisters causing itching). Right now I feel OK. These medical problems didn't really affect my functioning. But I do have to be careful with my back. Sometimes I slip a disc if I'm not careful. Doing my exercises really helps both physically and psychologically.

Coping with Having Had Cancer

Having the love and support of family and friends was the most important way I was able to cope with having cancer. Daily mindful-ness meditation (teaches one to slow down racing thoughts, be positive, and be calmed) was and continues to be a source of great comfort, hope, and getting my energy back. I was in a colon cancer support group at Gilda's Club for a time. People talked mostly about their treatment. Their stories were unique and heartbreaking. For some reason, I got more out of listening than I did out of sharing. Every-body was very supportive in the colon cancer group, but I wanted to hear about their emotional reactions to the cancer diagnosis and treatment. That was not done. Members of the group and I had bet-ter conversations in the parking lot. When we would leave the group session, people would then start talking about how they felt. I real-ized how lucky I was that I'm still alive. In addition, watching mov-ies, reading, exercising as much as I could, staying away from toxic situations as much as I could, seeing people with whom I felt com-fortable were all ways that I used to cope with having had cancer.

Satisfaction with Medical Care after Treatment and Through Survivorship

My oncologist is a wonderfully skilled and caring doctor, who always listens and enlists me as a partner in my treatment planning. I am relieved and grateful to know that these supports are there for me and my family. There is a system here of aftercare that is staffed by three nurses. Before you leave the hospital, one of these nurses comes in and asks if you would like to be called on a daily basis once you get home, to see how things are going. I did. When I got home from the hospital, the nurse called me every day for three weeks. I found myself waiting for the phone to ring or the nurse to call. Sometimes we would talk for an hour, an hour and a half. That gave me enormous physical and emotional support because I was able to talk about how I felt. This was superb, absolutely superb. I couldn't have asked for anything better.

Overall Impact of Having Had Cancer

Negative and Positive Effects

I am much less tolerant. I am too abrupt in responding to the questions of people who are struggling with cancer that I find intrusive. I am learning not to do that. I have become more in touch with my own kind of dumb things that I have said to people with medical problems. My intentions are always sincere and caring but how those concerns are shown can sometimes not be helpful. I am more and more aware of this.

Greatest Concerns

I have moved to a rental apartment so I need to sell my condo. I don't want my daughter to have to struggle with that after I'm gone. I worry about the world due to the pervasive rise of tyrants. I'm more concerned about that than having cancer.

Advice

Pay attention, ask questions, don't assume that the treatment team will explain things *(about the treatment)*. Be your own best advocate and don't assume you are asking a question that is not relevant, or have a silly reaction to something. Trust yourself! And last, peace, love, forgiveness.

KATHERINE W.: *Colon Cancer, disease stage not known, 86 years old, female, disease-free four years*

Quality of Life after Treatment and Through Survivorship

Regaining and/or Changing One's Life

I'm very, very lucky because I have had my colon taken out and did not have to have any other treatment whatsoever. I can't dwell on whether colon cancer comes back. I've got to dwell on how well I'm doing now. I'm a very active person. I'm very active in my church. I'm treasurer of my garden club, and I was on the board of a little theater here. I was on a lot of boards. I'm 86 years old, but I still keep going. There were no emotional, financial problems, other illnesses, or other stresses in my life. I'm very fortunate.

Relationships with Family, Friends, and Acquaintances

I've had lots of friends and lots of acquaintances that had cancer, with most having gotten through it. They have such a great attitude. They don't say, "Why me? Why me?" They just say, "You know what? This happened and I've got to live with it and we're going on with life as long as we can."

Overall Impact of Having Had Cancer

Greatest Concerns

I have children and great-grandchildren whom I'm very concerned about. I'm worried about them because I want them to be healthy and strong, that they will go the right road and have children.

Advice

I think faith is very important. I don't know how people get through with anything with no faith, no belief in God. He's going to take care of you whatever *(happens)*. My faith had gotten me through a lot of things in many years. About the only thing I can say is to have faith that you're going to get through it and you go on with your life. Hopefully, everybody will have as good an experience as I have had.

MARIE K.: *Colon Cancer, disease stage not known, 87 years old, female, disease-free five years*

Quality of Life after Treatment and Through Survivorship

Emotional State

They did a colonoscopy two years after surgery and everything turned out fine. That was my biggest worry.

Relationships with Family, Friends, and Acquaintances

My whole family was pulling for me, but my husband was the one that had to bear a lot of it. If I'm upset, he's upset. He's my partner. One of my friends just died last year, and I do miss her terribly, because she's the one you could talk to. She knew how you felt before you even said it. She understood, without my saying anything.

Other Non-Cancer Medical Problems and Stressful Events

I broke my pelvis and elbow two years ago. It can be very painful, but it wasn't. It healed. I called my son and about 20 minutes later he was able to come to our home. He wanted to see if I could go up the stairs. I knew how to do it. I got up and down the stairs, going on my butt all the way up and did it the same way coming down. It didn't hurt.

Overall Impact of Having Had Cancer

Greatest Concerns

I'm just trying to go from one day to another. I'm getting tired. It's a challenge being of the age I am now. My husband and I are both feeling that way. I'm finding every day a little bit more of a challenge, unfortunately.

Advice

If a patient has to take chemo, that is very hard. But now, cancer treatment has advanced so much, that I think a patient should ponder it—look for the silver lining. There's always a chance that everything will be OK.

Chapter 3

Older Survivors of
Non-Hodgkin Lymphoma

As 74,680 NHL (non-Hodgkin lymphoma) cancer patients were diagnosed in 2018, NHL became the seventh largest type of cancer when compared to all other types of cancer in the United States. Approximately 56.2% of NHL cancer patients were diagnosed with NHL when 65 years old or older, and the rate of survival of five years or more is 71.4% (National Cancer Institute, SEER Cancer Stat Facts). Those who were treated at an earlier disease stage (Stages I and II, Lower grade) often, but not always, have an easier treatment compared to those with more advanced disease (Stages III and IV, Higher grade).

Important research has been done concerning the quality of life of NHL survivors who have been followed a number of years after their diagnosis. Physical and mental health problems became worse in 25% of survivors who were 10 to 15 years after being diagnosed (Smith et al. 2013). In addition, social activities were found to be worse in NHL cancer survivors requiring treatment (Kim et al. 2012). Further, 25% of NHL survivors reported not being satisfied with their sexual life, with 26% saying that it was a moderate to big problem in their lives (Beckjord et al. 2011).

Many of the NHL participants reported having regained or changed what they wanted their life to be like after treatment, that would be at least partially or largely satisfying to them, even after having difficult treatments. However, for several participants, one of the side effects of treatment, peripheral neuropathy, made it difficult to regain the quality of life that they had before having

NHL. Peripheral neuropathy is a very painful side effect of several commonly used chemotherapy treatments for non-Hodgkin lymphoma, which limits many activities involving patients' hands or feet. Current treatments for peripheral neuropathy were not able to reduce the pain at all in one NHL participant. While peripheral neuropathy occurred in only two NHL survivors out of 13 NHL participants in this book, it is likely that it affects many NHL patients across the nation in their ability to cope with having had cancer. It is important to keep in mind that in addition to peripheral neuropathy, other side effects of treatment also occur, as well as other non-cancer problems, further affecting NHL cancer survivors' quality of life.

INTO AND THROUGH TREATMENT

FLNEWT: *NHL Mantle Cell Lymphoma, Stage IV, 67 years old, male, in remission two years*

Life One Year Before Diagnosis

I'm an environmental engineer, working for the county government in a waste water facility. I'm also a marathoner. I did a whole bunch of different marathons all around the country, beginning in 1977. I've also raised funds for the Leukemia and Lymphoma Society.

Diagnosis of NHL Mantle Cell Lymphoma

It was April 2014 when I had a shoulder problem. I also noticed about in January that I had a lump on my neck. I thought it was a giant cyst. I went to see my doctor about my shoulder. The doctor scheduled the lymph node analysis, and then I had a CT scan, a PET scan, a bone marrow biopsy, and a colonoscopy. They diagnosed it as mantel cell lymphoma. The cancer was everywhere. It was stage

IV. (*It was decided*)* to go with this new protocol of thalidomide and Rituxan.

Treatment and Treatment Side Effects

Thalidomide screwed my system up a lot. I ended up in the hospital for a week, so that the doctor could straighten everything out. Once I got past that first week, I was fine. After Thalidomide I was given Rituxan. I stopped taking Rituxan after two years of treatment. I was clearly in complete remission.

Quality of Life During Treatment

Emotional State

There was a little bit of concern, obviously. I knew in the back of my mind that it's potentially fatal, but I never really thought of it that way. I thought it was just another fight to get through and beat it. I am going to relapse at some point in time, but I'll deal with it when it comes. I had too many other things I wanted to do before I get out of here.

Relationships with Family, Friends, and Acquaintances

I think my family was concerned, but they didn't really display it. My wife never dreaded this whole thing. She was very supportive. When I had the Rituxan treatment at the cancer center, I just sat there and she'd be there with me the whole time. My sons and daughters, along with our grandkids, lived with us through our whole treatment process, helping to support my wife and I.

---

* *Italicized (slanted) typing is used in parentheses when quoting participants to complete their sentences, in order to make the quotes clearer.*

I had several friends who were cancer survivors or spouses of cancer survivors who helped me along the way. My friends treated me as they had before my diagnosis. I really felt no special treatment, which was important to me at work. No one said they were sorry for me and I really never dwelt on the issue.

Employment

Since I worked for the county government, I have a lot of sick time. I only used a week *(of being out sick)* and my coworkers, like my friends, treated me as before my diagnosis. I didn't have any issues with my boss *(about being out)*. I have one coworker who has gone through thyroid cancer, so she understood. It was encouraging. One interesting thing happened to me at work. I was in a meeting with a consultant and several coworkers. The consultant said he felt someone needed healing prayers. I spoke up about my cancer and the consultant had everyone place their hands on me, and he prayed. I think that helped me too.

Religion

It was a combination of religious beliefs that the church provides along with the comradery with the people that helped me cope— just knowing that God wasn't going to let me go. If you just go to church once a week and you don't participate in any way, you don't get the support that you would probably need. Being in marathons and knowing that you can finish it is just another test of endurance *(in addition to having mantle cell lymphoma)*.

Satisfaction with Medical Care During Treatment

The oncologist, healthcare team, and the quality of my care were all excellent. I was able to benefit from a just-completed clinical trial. The drug company waived the cost since I had Stage IV cancer.

LIL: *Large B Cell Lymphoma, disease stage not known, 69 years old, female, disease-free four years; Prior cancer: Uterine Leiomyosarcoma*

Life One Year Before Diagnosis

I have always been very active physically and professionally. Before my first cancer, a rare uterine leiomyosarcoma, I taught at a university, but I gave up my position to focus on my health as I'd been told I had at most three years to live. Before the second cancer, I continued to do a bike ride *(62 miles)*, and backpack and canoe in the wilderness in North America. Professionally, I continued to write books for young readers as well as articles and reviews for professional journals. I put my activist energy into cancer advocacy *(helping cancer patients)*.

Diagnosis of NHL

(The doctor's nurse said) "I have good news for you. You don't have a recurrence of leiomyosarcoma *(prior cancer with a poorer prognosis than non-Hodgkin lymphoma)*. You have non-Hodgkin lymphoma (NHL) and we know how to treat that one." This was such great news. I was a survivor of uterine leiomyosarcoma, which is a rare uterine cancer. Our biggest fear was a recurrence, for which there was no known treatment at that time. Because I have been working in the cancer world in a leadership position in a cancer organization in my community, I had a lot of friends who really understood what was going on.

Treatment and Treatment Side Effects

(With the initial treatment failing), my local, rural family doctor began an hour-long conversation, mostly a diatribe, about when to give up a good fight. My doctor had said that I had everything that modern medical medicine had to offer, but it then failed and that I needed to prepare to die. He said that survival was six months." I went into

this really deep depression. However, the doctor who did the stem cell transplant said, "Either your doctor knows something that we don't know, or he was sadly mistaken." Just the possibility of survival changed everything. What followed was a long period that included inpatient chemo at the medical center, surgical biopsy, and radiation to prepare me for transplant, which would then require two more months of in-hospital treatment. It was a hard and uncertain time. There were many setbacks. But my husband and I had done cancer before. He rented a room near the hospital. We dug in.

With R-CHOP *(chemotherapy regimen: rituximab, cyclophosphamide, doxorubicin, vincristine, prednisone)* and with later courses of chemo, I had all the usual side effects. Anti-nausea meds became my new best friends. I shaved my hair early on and adopted a bald pride attitude: This is my life now, why should I hide it?

Quality of Life During Treatment

Emotional State

If I had focused on the side effects I would have been miserable. So I focused on what I could do. Maybe I felt weak, but I could walk halfway around the pond in this local park, and then sit for half an hour, and then walk the other halfway around to the car. There were times when I couldn't do much, but I also had really good friends who would walk with me around the pond and sit and just look at the ducks and talk about stuff.

Relationships with Family, Friends, and Acquaintances

My doctor was not able to remove the tumor, so I had more treatment. The tumor didn't go away. It grew. That wasn't my worst time, but I think it was my husband's worst time. He left the lab that he founded and he was in the middle of research. I said *(to my husband)*, "You've got to take care of yourself. Go ride a bike," because I know that's what he does to take care of himself. He did. He rode his bike across the Golden Gate Bridge, and I heard him say, "It's a gorgeous, beautiful day." We watched dolphins beneath *(the bridge)*, ships are coming in and the wind was in my face, and then suddenly I said, "It's just so good to be alive." As much as possible we supported each other, but meeting his emotional needs was too much for me at times. I'm sure he felt the same way.

My sons being able to help me at various stages of having had cancer felt good. At various times through this whole saga, one or the other of my two sons would come and stay with me when I had surgery and going through stem cell transplant. They came a couple of times so that *(my husband)* could get some relief. That's important in taking care of a caregiver.

My friends were amazing, especially those who were dealing with cancer or had in the past. A former student of mine and now colleague, made a comforter that showed me cycling through hilly vineyards. I slept under that dream quilt in the transplant ward and I still treasure it.

Sexual Life

I decided that I was going to continue to have a sex life, despite everything that was happening to me. We both wanted to continue being close in that way, and we have, with some interruptions, like when I was in the hospital.

Coping with Having Cancer

I had support from my cancer organization, Humboldt Breast Health Project, and my friends were there. We had worked on a lot of stuff together, but I stopped volunteering in that way *(when diagnosed with NHL)*. My job became survival again.

One of the things I learned was how to accept help. That was a big deal to be able to do. "Yes. If you'd bring me some food that would be so fabulous." Somebody said to me early on in the first cancer *(leiomyosarcoma)*, "Don't rob your friends and family of the gift of helping you and being able to do something. They need that."

Satisfaction with Medical Care During Treatment

I went to a *(major cancer center)*. The medical team was outstanding. These were people at the forefront of research, but they were also very warm human beings. A fabulous research doctor who oversaw all my treatment, walked every step of the way with me through a lot of different steps to get to the stem cell cancer lab. My doctors felt like we were all in a team together. I really felt like *(my husband)* and I were equal players on the team with the different medical people who were involved. We all talked with each other comfortably, and they felt that we understood what they were talking about. For the stem cell transplant, I was on a ward with other people who were going to be there for a long period of time. It was a really well set-up, beautifully organized, beautifully staffed unit for people who were going through terrible things. There's tremendous strength that *(patients)* have to give to each other and indeed in the relationships that I did develop there *(during treatment)*. Some of these relationships continue to this day. We would gather in somebody's room or in the common room, and that was a real time of closeness with those who were going through this. There should have been more of those kinds of things—they would have helped me a whole lot. That's what this grassroots breast cancer organization did *(when I had the prior cancer, uterine leiomyosarcoma)*. It was all peer support, helping each other through having cancer. *(However, in the cancer center)*, there was only one one-hour support group, and the only people who came actually were men. We did have musicians come and play things for us. The music really brought us together and uplifted us.

ROY M.: *NHL, Grade 3, 70 years old, male, in remission one year*

Life One Year Before Diagnosis

My health was fine the year prior *(to my diagnosis)*. My wife's health was fine. We did not have financial issues, but things were not very fulfilling, probably more so for me than my wife. There just was not a lot of social engagement *(before we moved)*. There was a sense of isolation. *(When we moved)* there were huge changes in just the addition of so many friends and having a huge variety of things. It made my life so much more enriching and this cancer diagnosis so livable. I stopped working in the claims legal area *(the job before I)* took on a different role *(in my life)*. I taught high school and college kids to be lifeguards and I worked for the local YMCA *(gyms available nationwide)*. It really got me into a heightened awareness of the importance of fitness, which played a big part in my life since diagnosis. I had been diagnosed with dysthymic disorder *(persistent depression)* a while back, before my cancer diagnosis. I've battled that for years and have been taking Paroxetine since then. However, I have functioned at a high level, even with having depression.

Diagnosis of NHL

My physician ordered some tests done. I still remember getting the phone call saying, "You have lymphoma. You're going to be fine. You're fit. This has a significant cure rate. You're lucky you got this kind of cancer versus some other one." Getting that diagnosis just knocks you down. It wasn't a total surprise, but it started the whole string of reactions which so many of us go through: anger, denial, bouncing back and forth. I think that the toughest thing was the anger.

Treatment and Treatment Side Effects

At the time of the first treatment I was in good shape. The doctor said, "I expect you to do 70% of your activities, but don't do dumb things." He knew that I was a pretty avid bike rider. He pointed out the fatigue I was going to experience *(due to chemotherapy)* and was not the type that one can fight through, so don't try it *(going on a long bike ride)*." The hematologist said, "Here are your orders. Get with it." It's like when I was a medic in the army the year before my cancer diagnosis. "You've got your orders. This is what your mission is, and you do your damndest to accomplish it." I had 18 weeks of chemotherapy *(R-CHOP: rituximab, cyclophosphamide, doxorubicin, vincristine, prednisone)* and six three-week cycles. I did have some weight loss, and nausea, which was controlled. *(Out of all the treatments I had after this one)*, it really was the easiest. I wound up in complete remission. There was some fatigue, but I continued to do work, other than my going to the YMCA *(gym)*, and bike riding.

About two years later I again noticed lymph nodes popping up. The doctors at *(medical center)* found that I had an aggressive cancer with diffuse large B-cells. The doctor said: "Not bad, but you have an indolent form, Grade 3 follicular lymphoma." The treatment before the stem cell treatment was RICE *(rituximab, ifosamide, carboplatin, etoposide)*. That was nine more weeks of chemo. I don't recall it being any harsher than R-CHOP. I was able to continue to do things *(that I wanted to do)* like bike riding. The Lymphomaniacs is a local bike team used to raise monies for the Leukemia and Lymphoma Society *(charitable organization providing research, information, and support services for leukemia and lymphoma patients)*. Next year will be my fifth year of participating. It's a two-day ride, 75 miles per day. It's just one of the things that kept me sane.

The worst part of the stem cell transplant was RICE. After therapy ended, it got to be very tough. I think I lost 22 pounds. When I got home, I could not walk probably more than a couple hundred feet. For the nausea, you have to keep taking Zofran *(anti-nausea medication)*. It works for most people. It didn't work for me. With having no strength, *(and)* fatigue and nausea, it took a long time to recover. I think I am still recovering. But, it worked.

Quality of Life During Treatment

Emotional State

I think for any cancer patient, if you're angry as a person before having cancer, you'll probably have moments where you're even angrier
once you're diagnosed. I felt like that was me. It was not present all
the time, but it happened every now and then. After a number of
trips to the hospital, I'd get frustrated and angry, but, for the most
part, that went away once I think I truly accepted that I had cancer. However, that applied to the first treatment with R-CHOP. That
anger probably came back after the stem cell transplant.

Relationships with Family, Friends, and Acquaintances

I think that the toughest thing was the anger. I pushed that anger
onto my wife. That's been in our marriage for a long time. *(However)*, my wife's caring has gotten me through *(my having had cancer)*.
She was just a steadfast presence for me at the hospital, every day.
Fortunately, I was very fit at the start of both of the chemotherapy
treatments, R-CHOP and RICE. But, after I got home from the
transplant, I couldn't do a whole lot. She took up all the slack. My
wife took care of meds, driving me to the medical appointments
when I could not drive, and getting adult diapers for me due to
the unbelievable diarrhea. That was caused by the transplant with
RICE before it. I was pretty antisocial after the transplant—I felt so
cruddy. But, I did have a couple of my good friends from the biking
team. I have another friend who is an 18-year survivor of multiple
myeloma, which is unheard of. He went through pretty much the
same thing I had. I was trying to cast a net as widely as I could to
people that had been through *(what I had)*. They gave me perspective.

My son was so supportive—just checking in *(to see how I was
doing)*, or coming over. He did bike rides with me and supported the

fundraising efforts of the Leukemia and Lymphoma Society. What has been most helpful for my wife were friends that we've met since we moved here. She also has gotten great support from her son and daughter-in-law.

Coping with Having Cancer

When we moved into a condo which has 320 homes, there was just a great mix of people that reached out to us. They told us in the first days *(after I was diagnosed with having lymphoma)* about Gilda's Club *(organization that provides services for cancer patients)*. We immediately went there. In our support group at Gilda's Club, if a new member came in, one of the guys in the group would say "You're going to like this place because cancer is spoken here and nobody has a problem with it." Both of us have friends there that we do things with. I think that has been so healthy for both my wife and myself. *(In fact),* overall, the biggest things that helped me get past the pain of diagnosis were probably a combination of support groups at Gilda's Club and some really good medical information. I would go to the medical school library and they will print anything that you want for free. Lots of cancer patients I've talked to do not want this information, but then they have got to have an advocate that can do it for them.

Institutionalized religion did not play a role in helping me cope with having cancer. While we raised our son we went to church, but now have totally drifted away. For me I fully agree with people who believe that spirituality is beneficial. For me, thoughts about accepting this diagnosis, accepting doubt, accepting our being mortal, brought courage to me.

Satisfaction with Medical Care During Treatment

I had a great doc. He set realistic expectations. The nurses were so helpful when I was in the hospital getting chemotherapy. The best oncologists and hematologists realize that you can be cured once in a while, and can alleviate suffering often. But the best oncologists and nurses are compassionate, and I thought they were as a group. I think that's important for good care. But, as a patient, you have to do your part. The good Lord helps those who help themselves. I think that it helps to have that attitude.

STEVE: *NHL, Stage I, 70 years old, male, in remission one year*

Life One Year Before Diagnosis

I had never been sick in my life. I was an incredibly active person. I did extremely difficult physical exercises every day. I volunteered at the San Diego Zoo three days a week. Rode my bike everywhere. Our marriage was getting a little bit better since we moved to San Diego. I just love talking to the people and meeting people from all over the world. I've had Attention Deficit/Hyperactivity Disorder (ADHD) since childhood. ADHD is just a horrible thing. My whole life I had trouble in school and getting along with people. I have difficulty staying on the subject and my mind wanders. If I go to a movie, you ask me four days later, I won't be able to tell you very much about that movie at all. I never remembered how to do anything. It was really difficult and frustrating for me—it affected my whole life.

Diagnosis of NHL

I felt something weird in one of my testicles. There was this hardness feeling. The testicle was removed. The pain in my legs was so unbelievable. Younger people who talked about this on the internet said that they had similar pain problems for three or four weeks and then they started getting much better. My pathology report showed a low-grade non-Hodgkin lymphoma. The hardest thing that I found from the minute I started this ordeal was that I couldn't find other men my age on the internet who were going through what I was going through. I tried so hard just to find anybody to talk to about what they're experiencing.

Treatment and Treatment Side Effects

The testicle was removed. The treatment made me unbelievably sick. I just didn't leave the apartment very much. *(I had relapsed on four different treatments)*. When I was done with the bone marrow transplant *(one of the treatments)*, you're basically dead. I was very tired and could hardly move and I had terrible pain from peripheral neuropathy. It lasted at least one month. It was awful, but I survived it. I forced myself to go into the pool maybe a week after the transplant. Doing my little aerobic stuff in the pool has been one of the things that kept me going. I had terrible skin problems throughout *(all the different treatments)*. Lyrica *(medication to treat neuropathic pain)* destroyed my skin. Flexeril *(medication to treat muscle spasms)* was unbelievable. I tried everything. During those days I was open to trying anything for my pain, and nothing changed it.

Quality of Life During Treatment

Emotional State

I've always been positive. I always felt that I was going to get better. I just said "OK, I've got to deal with this; it is what it is." I had a testicle removed. I'm in a lot of pain. I got depressed. I did cry many times in the first couple of years when I was feeling so bad. Now I've got to go forward and try and handle the situation. That's the way I looked at it at that point in time. I never let fear destroy me. The hardest thing when you have this disease is just dealing with the unknown.

Relationships with Family, Friends, and Acquaintances

When we moved here, I was starting to make friends, but that all ended abruptly when I got sick. I couldn't do anything anymore because I was so sick all the time from the treatments. *(However, there was)* a cancer patient in my building and we would just sit and talk. He would tell me what he had been going through his whole life. I talked about myself. We had a real friendship.

I think people are afraid of people who have cancer. They don't know what to say to them. That is one of the worst things that you have to deal with when you're a cancer patient. Other people, when they look at you, you start to get this feeling—*(they're thinking)* "Can I catch it from him by being this close?" It's just awful and you just feel so different from other people.

Satisfaction with Medical Care During Treatment

I went to an oncologist who my friend, who I really trust, *(had recommended)*. This first doctor was just the nicest man in the world. The problem was that he was incompetent. The second doctor—he had no feeling for patients. It was like I was a burden to him. I would question him. He didn't like it a bit. We didn't get along very well. The third doctor, got me the very last slot in a clinical trial designed to treat my neuropathy which caused such terrible pain due to the chemo. She convinced me that if I didn't do another bone marrow biopsy and PET scan I would be hurting her by abandoning the protocol. These tests only brought me more pain. The fourth doctor—I love her. I trust her emphatically with my life. She's just got this ability to relate to people and you know she cares about you and talks to you realistically. At the hospital I was going to at that time, I was put in a big room and you felt like cattle in there. But the nurses were fantastic. I wouldn't be alive without the oncology nurses that I was fortunate to have by my side over the last five years. The doctors don't have enough time for patients. The oncology nurses are the ones that keep you going.

RON: *NHL, Burkitt's Lymphoma, Stage IV, 72 years old, male, disease-free four years*

Life One Year Before Diagnosis

The year before I was diagnosed, I just ended a three-year divorce. It was a horrible divorce. Outside of that, I was playing tennis tournaments. I was in incredible physical condition. There were no signs of any cancer. After the divorce, I went on with my life and I had a wonderful girlfriend—still have the same girlfriend.

Diagnosis of NHL

I have a wonderful friend that's been in acupuncture. My symptoms, which were basically my bowel *(movements)*, were jet black and oozing. *(My friend)* started yelling at me to get into the ER immediately. She recognized that that there was something internally that was completely wrong. I went to the ER and the doctor told me that I had cancer. "You have what's called Burkitt's lymphoma, and it's the fastest growing cancer that we know of. Chemo works really good against it."

Treatment and Treatment Side Effects

The doctors just basically chemoed me out for three weeks, after they had first hydrated me. You get delirious, especially after being hydrated at 163 degrees. The biggest side effect was probably all the coughing. I couldn't stop coughing and I ended up losing my voice for two months. *(The coughing)* was probably the most aggravating thing of the whole deal. My girlfriend is into essential oils *(to treat the coughing)*, and really helped me out with that. That made a huge difference. *(However)*, the most painful things were the things *(the doctors did)* to check out what was causing these *(problems, such as)* putting a hose down my nose and throat. You lose your taste buds for the most part. Food really became bland, with the exception of ice cream, fruits, and sweets, which tasted good. The worst procedure was the lumbar puncture, to draw the liquid out of your spine and then replace that liquid with chemo. I had five of those *(one month apart)*. By the time they got to the fourth *(lumbar puncture)*, there wasn't any liquid in my spine to pull out. So, they would try and change positions of the needle to pull it out, and when it hit that nerve, it would just have a tremendous shock effect going right down your leg. The fourth *(lumbar puncture)* was bad, but the fifth one was just out of control.

(Due to significant weight loss, the nutritionist said,) "You need to eat anything and everything and as much as you want. You've got to get your weight up. Start working out again." So, after that session, I started working out like crazy again. My son took me over to get medical marijuana, which would make me hungry.

Quality of Life During Treatment

Emotional State

And then you go on with doing your thing and let *(the doctor)* do his thing and you hope everything comes out okay. That relaxed me. I would chant, I would just basically say, "I've had a wonderful life. Everybody dies." If this is my time to die, I can honestly say that I don't owe anybody anything. I'm financially stable, the kids are both self-sufficient and my girlfriend has been just absolutely wonderful through the whole procedure, and that's it. Everything is being done that can be done. So, it's out of my hands entirely, so why fret over it?

Relationship with Family, Friends, and Acquaintances

My girlfriend was an angel; she was incredible. She's Filippina. Filippinos have a smile on their face—they're very positive. No negativity whatsoever. And that's the way she handled the whole thing. I don't know if I could have done what she did.

My brother and my best friend were at the hospital when all the chemo treatments were being done. A lot of my fraternity brothers came over. Most of the driving back and forth to the hospital was done by my tennis friend, who also had melanoma and skin cancer. Even when he was going through all of that, he was driving me. One guy came from 40 miles away, picked me up, took me to *(the medical center)*. So, I had all my friends entered into the equation. I had prayer vigils going on. Learning how much they really cared for me—that's what got me emotionally.

Coping with Having Cancer

I just gave myself to the Lord. I knew I was surrounded by the best of the best: best friends, best doctors, best family, and best caring girlfriend. There were all kinds of prayer vigils and I did a lot of praying on my own. I said "I had a wonderful life, I have two incredible kids." I took all the worry away from myself and put the responsibility on the doctors and the Lord. I said, "If it is to be, it'll work out." *(The Lord)* will give the doctors the wherewithal to make the right decisions and I'll live. And, if it's not to be, I'll pass on, but with a free conscience.

Satisfaction with Medical Care During Treatment

(The medical care) was wonderful. *(My oncologist)* is the sweetest person I could have been with. She's incredible.

KAYE C.: *NHL, disease stage not known, 74 years old, female, disease-free 2.5 years*

Life One Year Before Diagnosis

Things were going *(well)*, other than tremendous fatigue. My family was good. My kids were good. My husband was a rock. I have some wonderful friends. We have four grandboys and two grandgirls. They were amazing. I love them to pieces. That's what I did for a year before my diagnosis. I did everything I always did. I've been a very healthy person. We led a very good life.

Diagnosis of NHL

I noticed a complete lack of energy—tremendous fatigue. I had no inkling that I had cancer. The doctor sent me to an oncologist who sent me to *(the medical center)* for a biopsy, where I was finally diagnosed with lymphoma of the central nervous system. My relationship with my family was still very good.

Treatment and Treatment Side Effects

I had six months of chemotherapy before the stem cell transplant, where I was in the hospital for four days every two weeks getting chemo. After that I was able to get my stem cell transplant. I think the most painful part of it was when I had an eye biopsy. Other than that I wasn't in much pain at all. *(The medical center)* was just wonderful. They were very concerned about that. My only real complaint was the fatigue and weakness. Losing my hair wasn't a problem. A couple of friends made me hats and scarves. Prior to losing my hair, I went and got a wig. When I went out in public I wore the wig. That didn't bother me.

Quality of Life During Treatment

Emotional State

I was very hopeful and energized. *(The medical center)* was very encouraging. They said statistically stem cell transplants are very, very effective and that I was doing very well. I thought I was too.

Relationships with Family, Friends, and Acquaintances

My friends were all just wonderful. When I was through with my stem cell transplant, we had a party for them to thank them for all they did. My husband took over and my friends did too. They were just wonderful. They sent food over often. They visited often. They helped my husband tremendously. I'll never be able to repay them. If my husband didn't feel I should be left alone, occasionally *(my friends)* would come over and grocery shop, cleaned my house one day, and just did all kinds of things. I can't thank them enough.

Coping with Having Cancer

No question about it, I got the help I needed from *(the medical center)*. I was very encouraged that this was going to be taken care of. Coping was not a problem—it really wasn't.

Satisfaction with Medical Care During Treatment

I was tremendously satisfied. My oncologist was on top of it and explained everything.

MARSHA JEAN LUNDMARK: *NHL, Stage I, 77 years old, female, disease-free 2.5 years*

Life One Year Before Diagnosis

Everything seemed normal. I am retired, my husband is retired, but we are very active. I really have had very good health all of my life.

There was nothing that happened that would make me wonder if something was wrong.

Diagnosis of NHL

In December of 2014 I had my annual physical. My doctor noticed that my right tonsil had swelled a little. I hadn't noticed it because I didn't feel any different when I swallowed and didn't have a sore throat. But after that, on occasion, I would look in my throat. By March, I noticed that my right tonsil had swelled more and it looked like I had little blisters all over me. It was really kind of ugly. So I called and made an appointment with my doctor. She looked at it and didn't have any idea what it was, so she made an appointment for me to see an ear, nose, and throat doctor. He took a biopsy of it, and it came back negative. The doctor said he didn't really like the looks of it and said, if it was alright with me, he would take another biopsy and try to get further scrapings and sent it in again. It still came back negative, and he said "I can take your tonsils out or I can send this biopsy to Florida where they do further testing." I said, "That's fine with me." So he did that, and it came back that it was lymphoma. They discovered that there were two different kinds of lymphoma and one was more aggressive than the other. He therefore wanted me to see an oncologist. A bone marrow biopsy was done, which came back negative. I then had a PET scan, which showed that the cancer was only in that right tonsil. It wasn't in any other place in my body. I am very thankful that my doctor was so persistent. However, because they had to send the biopsy to Florida, it took a long time to be analyzed. That was stressful. I didn't know what was going to happen. It was worse than knowing something and facing it. I was kind of relieved to know *(that I had lymphoma)* and that I can be treated. The cancer doctors I dealt with were extremely compassionate. They made you feel at ease and told you everything that was going on. When I was reading my devotions for that day, there was a verse in Isaiah 41 that said, "Don't be afraid, I am with you. I am your God, let nothing terrify you. I will make me strong and I will protect you and sit with you." I haven't been afraid; it was what I needed. I still carry that verse with me.

Treatment and Treatment Side Effects

I had three chemo treatments *(CHOP: cyclophosphamide, doxorubi-cin, vincristine, prednisone)*. After I had the second chemo treatment, you could tell that looking at my tonsil, the swelling was going down. I had the third treatment, and then had another PET scan. It showed that my tonsil was all clear. Because there were two kinds of non-Hodgkin lymphoma, they wanted me to have the 15 radiation treatments, just to make sure. So I had 15 radiation treatments. The PET scan again showed that I was cancer-free. When I had the radiation, it made my throat sore after a while. I had trouble eating and lost a few pounds. It took a while for that to go away. I was very tired, mostly during the chemotherapy—I really felt beat. I think it was really over when the treatments were over. With the chemo, I would also get a little nauseous once in awhile, and of course, my hair fell out after three weeks of the first treatment. It was yucky. The Zonta Club *(provides services to women and children)* gives anybody who had lost their hair a wig. With a wig, nobody would know because I basically looked the same way when I had my hair. It really didn't bother me to let people know that I had cancer. But, I didn't want to be different *(because I was wearing a wig)*, with people saying, "Look at her, look at her hair." Some people didn't even know *(that I had a wig)* until I told them. They said, "Oh really, I didn't notice." The wig did its job.

Quality of Life During Treatment

Functioning

I never missed a Sunday at church. Sometimes I didn't feel the greatest, but I was always there. The doctors had told me that when my white count was low, not to go to a restaurant or do grocery shopping. They didn't want you to put yourself in contact with any germs that you would pick up from others. One Friday night we were going out with my husband's brother and wife for dinner. Because my blood count was low, we picked up our food from the restaurant and went to the park instead of the restaurant. That was supportive too.

Relationships with Family, Friends, and Acquaintances

It was mostly just my husband who helped me. I did have a few days sporadically when I didn't feel great. When I had the long chemo treatments and I'd sit for six to eight hours having medications going into me, he was always with me. If I couldn't do something at home or fix a meal, he did that. I have a son and a daughter, and they were always supportive and wanted to be on top of what was happening. One time, when I was having a treatment and I didn't know it was going to be a long one, and I was taking a long time to get back home, my daughter was calling and wondering where I was. She was very concerned and wondering if everything was OK. My oldest grandson called all the time, always wondering how I was and being supportive. My three granddaughters were still at home, working here, always wondering how Grandma was. My family has always been connected closely with our church and our faith. I have a lot of friends at church, and they were all very supportive and concerned, always wanting to know how things were going. That was very helpful. It meant a lot. However, I think it was because I wasn't afraid of having lymphoma, and I felt strong, that I only needed to keep my family in touch with what was being done and how I felt. They just felt OK because I was OK. Friends were all concerned and supportive.

Coping with Having Cancer

God helped me cope with being treated for cancer. He showed me several places in the Bible where it says, "Don't be afraid." I keep finding more and more verses that said that. Also, when I go to these doctors' offices, and they are full of people who are worse off than you are, I felt very fortunate that my cancer was found when it was just a little more than Stage I.

Satisfaction with Medical Care During Treatment

I was very satisfied with the medical care. I am very happy with the doctors, from my own personal physician, to the ear, nose, and throat doctor, and the two chemo doctors who I dealt with. Because my doctors saw my tonsil and because my ear, nose, and throat doctor was so persistent, they were able to identify lymphoma at an earlier stage. I was very, very happy with them.

ART B.: *NHL, Stage II, 80 years old, male, disease-free four years; Prior cancer: Acute Myeloid Leukemia (AML)*

Life One Year Before Diagnosis

I was diagnosed with AML (acute myeloid leukemia) in February 2007. For three years I was in remission and doing extremely well. In July 2008, my wife died of breast cancer. Though I did date a few women throughout this period, this effort had no potential for long term or intimate relationships. My thinking was that the leukemia diagnosis indicated that I didn't have much time left, so no one I met was willing to risk a relationship.

Diagnosis of NHL

In January 2011, I was being treated for kidney stones. The CT scan showed an enlarged lymph node, which was diagnosed after biopsy to be follicular lymphoma. I was annoyed. I had no symptoms. I was concerned that waiting might place me in a position of being too old for treatment, so I selected treatment. I said, "Well, I've got to do this."

Treatment and Treatment Side Effects

The treatment for follicular lymphoma is so easy by comparison *(to AML, prior cancer)*. I did all the normal things I would have done except for the day I went to get chemo. The chemo took a day and then I'd go home and do my normal things. I wasn't tired. I didn't have any side effects from any of the medications.

Quality of Life During Treatment

Emotional State

During treatment, going to the office for chemo monthly for several months seemed to be a bother. I re-evaluated my thinking because I recognized that if I wasn't enthusiastic about recovery I might miss an important treatment option. I have now learned that a second treatment would not be as effective as the first one. I'm not concerned because I made the best decision I could at the time. With my treatment, the stats showed no recurrence for at least 96% for seven years. I'm still one of the 96%.

Relationships with Family, Friends, and Acquaintances

My wife knew that I had lymphoma and wanted to go out with me anyway *(was dating her at that time)*. It's been generally a very, very good relationship. Most of the people I had asked to go out with me *(at that time)*, when they heard I had lymphoma, would run away like you wouldn't believe. I did tell people I had lymphoma because I found that sometimes somebody else has had a similar disease and by seeing my recovery going well, it gave them hope.

I think partly I minimized that I had NHL for my children. I didn't want to make it sound like I am dying, so you've got to come and see me. Sometimes I send them copies of what I write. I put it in a booklet on death and dying. I use that a lot with my friends. It shows my perspective on dying which is that I am going to live until I die. I'm not going to sit here and say: "Oh my God, I'm going to die." I know I'm going to die but I don't have to focus on that.

Coping with Having Cancer

I started thinking that the diagnosis was an annoyance. Then I realized that if I considered it an annoyance, I wouldn't treat myself properly. I said, "I've got to do this." So, I treated the diagnosis as important.

Satisfaction with Medical Care During Treatment

I believe that my doctor's expertise, her willingness to go beyond protocol, and her knowledge of leading edge research, has given me my life. *(However),* the (urology) surgeon didn't know that a needle biopsy wasn't good enough to diagnose lymphoma. There was no place in that treatment phase where questions were not answered. Even in the infusion center, the nurses there who were doing the infusions were very knowledgeable. I keep reading that doctors don't spend enough time with patients. I haven't found those doctors.

My community is one-tenth the size of San Jose *(had moved to San Rafael from San Jose),* so you can't expect to have the same level of treatment. I see how difficult it is for people who lived in small communities to survive these illnesses. This one guy I spoke to in Montana has to go to Seattle to get treated.

JUDY M.: *NHL, Stage II, 80 years old, female, disease-free three years*

Life One Year Before Diagnosis

For years I was a volunteer with the American Cancer Society. I had done a lot of work with them mostly in education, giving talks to groups, kids, civic groups about cancer, how they could look for *(cancer),* and avoid it. I was also very busy with my family and activities in my church. I was in the church choir, setting up the altar, washing the linens, and in a Bible study group. One year before I was diagnosed with non-Hodgkin lymphoma, my daughter was leaving her husband. We had to help her find another place to live. There was stress from that. During this time I was going for rehab for my knee and that was keeping me busy. I also had GERD *(gastroesophageal reflux disease)* which ended up with my having Barrett's esophagus and a hiatal hernia *(part of the stomach bulges into the chest, which may cause severe heartburn)*. I've been dealing with this for the year before my having cancer.

Diagnosis of NHL

For several years, I was having more and more trouble with my knee when walking. I had physical therapy; nothing worked, and it was still painful. I went to the doctor and he said, "I guess it's time to give you a knee replacement." I had a total knee replacement. I got a call from the orthopedic surgeon who said, "We discovered that you have cancer and it was a large B-cell lymphoma and non-Hodgkin lymphoma."

I happened to know of a group of oncologists because I was a volunteer with the American Cancer Society. So I immediately called to talk to one of the doctors. My main idea was, "Let's just get this thing taken care of." That's how I felt about it: go in, get done whatever has to be done and get rid of it, and that was my attitude. I pretty much stuck with that the whole time. I was anxious and fearful because you don't know what to expect and you don't know how it's going to turn out. My husband was concerned and upset about it. He agreed with me: "Let's just get to the doctor and an oncologist as soon as possible, and get something done about it." I went to see the oncologist *(at my medical center)* and had a PET scan. It showed that I had lymphoma, not only in my knee, but also in two lymph nodes in my groin. I was set up for a round of treatment.

Treatment and Treatment Side Effects

I had chemo *(treatment regimen)*, R-CHOP *(Rituxan, cyclophospha-mide, doxorubicin, vincristine, prednisone)*. It was going to get six treatments every three weeks. I felt tired and had a sore throat due to Rituxan, and constipation. I also had to take these other medications with R-CHOP. One was an antifungal and a couple more of anti-nausea medications. Then I had to take prednisone for five days. I had frequent urination at the beginning, because all that fluid going into you is going to come back out. Then, right before my next infusion, I started losing my hair. It was pretty devastating with the hair coming out and you can't do anything about it. I bought a wig and started wearing it. I was not going to *(go around)* being bald—it wouldn't be too pleasant to look at me. About the third infusion I started getting itchy in my armpits. Then I got a rash under my breast and I started getting little pustules coming out of my arm. One of the medicines I was taking was Diflucan. It was an anti-fungal medicine and that seemed to be causing the rashes and itching. It was pretty intense for a while. I couldn't sleep. I got some itch cream and that helped some, but it didn't do the job completely. I stopped using Diflucan and eventually the rash and itching went away.

When I felt weak and tired, I slept more than I normally did and took naps in the afternoon. Sometimes I couldn't sleep. I was still constipated throughout the whole thing. I felt like, "What's going to happen and how long is this going to drag on?" even though I knew it was only six rounds of chemo. I felt pretty good after we got the results in March that the cancer was gone.

Quality of Life During Treatment

Emotional State

Overall, it was kind of an up-and-down thing. There had been good times when I felt great, but there were times when I didn't.

Functioning

There may have been a period of time when I didn't feel great, so I didn't do some things. Sometimes I was too tired to do the shopping, and someone would go to the store and that was fine. But I tried to keep up with all the things I had been doing. I felt that doing this was good because then I wouldn't just dwell on the cancer. There really weren't *(any activities that I wanted to do but couldn't).*

Relationships with Family, Friends, and Acquaintances

My husband was very concerned about how I felt and how I was doing. He was very supportive. He drove me everywhere and stayed with me at all of the appointments. My children were concerned. They called and checked in with us to see how we were doing, how I was doing. Of course, most of them are far away. The only one nearby was my son in New Jersey. One's in England and the other one was out in Seattle. I didn't keep it a secret that I had cancer. I felt that it would better if everybody knew about it because they would then know what to look for if they had any problems themselves.

Coping with Having Cancer

I think probably what helped me the most was my background and my volunteer work with the American Cancer Society because I had been exposed to a lot of different people with different kinds of cancer. I ran a transportation group for a while where we would take people with cancer for their treatments. I saw different people in different stages of their treatments, and their attitudes in how they handled it. Considering the patients I saw, including myself, I thought if you have a positive attitude, you'll have a better outcome. I felt that being exposed to all the problems that I had over the years helped me to realize, "We're just going to do this. We're going to cope with whatever we have to *(due to cancer)*, and see what happens on the other end."

Satisfaction with Medical Care During Treatment

My doctor was fabulous. He took his time and explained things. The nurses were helpful and understanding and explained all the different medications I would be getting. I found that the nurses in the infusion room were just terrific. They'd help you out with anything you needed. They would bring in cookies and cakes for patients. I think that oncology is a field where if they go into this, they really are caring people. They have such a hard thing to deal with.

I would ask questions, whereas I think a lot of people don't know how to ask questions of the doctor. You have to know what to ask him. I think that helps. Most doctors would be willing *(to answer questions)*, but a lot of people just don't ask questions of their doctors. They accept whatever they're told. My doctor explained the outcome of what it would be and the percentage of people who had this cancer. He wrote it all out on a piece of paper for me.

PERL: *NHL, Stage IIIA, 81 years old, male, in remission 2.5 years*

Life One Year Before Diagnosis

I was in good health. I was doing all of the things that I do. We were doing things with our friends, riding the Harley-Davidson *(motorcycle)*, playing cards, fishing, walking in the winter, cross-country skiing, and doing everything that we love doing. We have four children and my wife is a wonderful lady, and we've been happy for 57 years. Everything was just fine until I noticed this growth.

Diagnosis with NHL

I went for my annual physical, and said to the doctor "I think I have a hernia." The doctor looked at it and said "I think you have a growth in there." In four days he called me and told me I had cancer—non-Hodgkin lymphoma. The word "cancer" scared the hell out of me. I was dumbfounded. I said, "I can't have cancer." But the doctor said, "It's one of the most curable cancers that you would have gotten." That gave me a little relief. After I was diagnosed, I would lie in bed and think about it. "How long do I have to live? What is going to happen and how is my family going to react?" I didn't get real depressed. I had a very positive attitude and I said, "We're going to beat this." I prayed a lot.

Treatment and Treatment Side Effects

Every three weeks after chemo, I'd be down for about five days. I couldn't do a lot—my body couldn't take it. After five days my body started repairing again and gave me a little bit more strength. By the end of three weeks, when I was about to go to the next chemo treatment, I was feeling pretty darn good. Then I got slammed down again.

Quality of Life During Treatment

Functioning

I was a member of the YMCA. I couldn't work like I wanted to, but I showed up five days a week when I could and did what I could to keep my body at least working. I wanted to keep my lifestyle as close to what I had before I was diagnosed.

Relationships with Family, Friends, and Acquaintances

My wife helped a lot. She's very positive about life and she is the same as I am as far as being a believer. She said, "We'll get through this." (*The chemotherapy*) did affect my sexual life. I couldn't perform for quite a while after that year when my body was recovering from the treatments. It took me a long time, but we're 80 years old—there's not a lot of a sexual life anyhow. But I guess there still is, but you slow down. My wife was very understanding. She's a professional nurse and she understands more than you would if someone had cancer.

My friends were shocked when I explained to them that I was diagnosed with cancer. My friends are all in the prayer groups that

I'm in, and they said, "We're going to do all we can to help you." A lot of my friends came up during chemotherapy and they sat with me. They gave me a lot of support—that meant so much to me—made me feel great. They tried to understand *(what I was going through)*, but they can't unless they actually went through it themselves. They did the best they could to keep me positive.

Religion

I'm not a real religious person but we go to church every Sunday. I am a strong believer. I did an awful lot of praying during my downtime with cancer. I had prayer groups at our church that were praying for me also. A lot of my relations sent me novenas *(special prayers and services)* about getting better and that helped me a lot.

Satisfaction with Medical Care During Treatment

(My oncologist) did a wonderful job. I had wonderful nurses at this cancer center. Some of them have had cancer, and they would tell me what they had gone through with chemo. It sure helped that I was talking to people who had cancer. It made me feel so good that they're in remission. I said, "I'm going to do the same thing." I got everything that I needed that was necessary to treat the cancer that I had *(in the cancer center in my home town)*. I talked to people that had been to these other cancer centers and when I told my friends I was going to be treated *(in my home town)*, they said, "Why do you want to do that? Why don't you go to a bigger town?" I said, "Because I'm getting the same treatment that I would have here, and I have faith in these people." They had all the facilities and the expertise that I needed to get through this traumatic time. A lot of people don't have faith in their local facility, but I do.

BARBARA G.: *NHL, Stage IV, Grade 1–2, 85 years old, female, in remission two years*

Life One Year Before Diagnosis

I've been healthy. I went to an exercise class every morning; I belong to two book groups and a writing group; I go to many of the courses in the Learning in Retirement program run by the college here; I am active in my church. So life was good.

Diagnosis of NHL

I had a blood test with my normal visit to my doctor and she noticed that my white blood cell count was low but it wasn't alarmingly low. I had another blood test three months later and the white blood cell count had decreased, so she sent me to a hematologist/oncologist during that year. He set up a bone marrow test which indicated that I had lymphoma. I didn't have any symptoms other than the blood test results. I got tired easily, but I was getting older and I assumed that was why. *(When I heard the diagnosis)*, I was very surprised, and not happy too. I think I was sort of numb and I accepted that I had lymphoma, but there must have been a little bit of denial, that it couldn't be happening to me. We all know how we are going to end up sometime, and cancer is scary.

(Both of my daughters) were quite upset. Cancer is something that you don't expect to end up well. My younger daughter worked as a chaplain in a hospital and she sent me a lot of information. I think maybe she was even more upset than I was because she knew that all of the possibilities were not necessarily good ones. She didn't upset me, she just tried to help educate me and boost me.

Treatment and Treatment Side Effects

Every Wednesday for four weeks, I would go in and have the chemotherapy. I would be kind of wiped out that day because it took several hours to do that. I didn't have any side effects from the chemotherapy—no nausea, hair loss, or anything like that. It was just tiring sitting there. Some lymph nodes were removed from my lungs, but some were still in my lungs, effects of the lymphoma, but it hasn't affected me. I didn't have trouble breathing. *(My oncologist)* explained to me that I was not going to get rid of the lymphoma, but it could be kept under control. I almost stopped going to the exercise class entirely. I'd at least went to exercise class in the morning for an hour class. Eventually, I was able to go to that full-time.

In March of 2016 I had a CT scan and it showed that the lymphoma was coming back stronger. So, I had a second series of chemotherapy, and again it was four Wednesdays in a row. Then everything was fine again.

Quality of Life During Treatment

Emotional State

I think in the beginning it was hard to accept what it was. I was overwhelmed and not totally accepting because it just seemed so far out. I had been healthy for so long that I couldn't imagine my getting cancer. As the hospital gave me some material to read as well as my daughter, I had read enough to understand what lymphoma was. So, gradually, I accepted the fact that that was the case with me—I had it. But it was just four weeks of treatment and such good results that I felt much better. The fear went away and all was well.

The second time that I needed to go through it, I knew what was going to happen and I think I expected the results again would be a good one. *(My oncologist)* had already told me that I would always have lymphoma. He did tell me that that's probably not what would kill me in the end, that it could be under control and that's okay with me.

Relationships with Family, Friends, and Acquaintances

Both of my daughters, on occasion, went with me when I had the treatment. The daughter that lives with me has been supportive and anything I asked her to do for me, she did. She was able to physically help me where my younger daughter, who lives in Idaho, could only verbally do that. My younger daughter came to visit during the second round of treatment and went in with me, stayed with me. That made me feel good. I think maybe it was reassuring to *(both daughters)* too, to see that there wasn't something horrible happening. When you hear chemo you expect the worst, but it wasn't anything that hurt. It was just kind of tedious and they saw how well I was looked after *(at the medical center)*. One of my longtime friends who went with me while I had a test to determine whether or not it was lymphoma was very supportive. She is one of the most intelligent persons that I know and she was able to talk to me about lymphoma. Just being supportive I could sense a big change *(in me)*.

Religion

I regularly attend church and I have a strong belief in God. My church family cared about my health and let me know that. They prayed for me. I do believe in the power of prayer and felt comfortable with their attention. I've done a number of Bible studies, I use a devotional book every morning, and church is a very important part of my life. A good number of my close friends are ones that I have met in church. I do believe in the power of prayer. I don't think that every prayer is answered with a "Yes." Some of them get a "No." But I do pray and it was helpful to me while I was having the cancer treatment. My close friends in church had been very supportive. They've asked about how I am doing and are happy to hear when things are going well. At church we have what's called a prayer chain *(group of people who pray together)*, and anyone can ask to be put on it or be put on it by someone else if they are having a medical or any kind of a problem. Then there are 30 to 35 people alerted to that and asked to pray for that person.

Satisfaction with the Medical Care During Treatment

I liked my oncologist very much. I trust him and I find him to be encouraging. He is willing to answer my questions and I am glad that he is the person who is treating my lymphoma. The people in the cancer clinic at the hospital I go to are wonderful people. They are kind and they are truly concerned with patients and they don't give you the feeling that they are in a hurry. One of the nurses that worked in the lab where I had the treatment was wonderful. Most of the times that I would go in she would be the one dealing directly with me. She was very attentive. I would get cold while I was having the treatment and she would bring a warm blanket, anything I needed to drink. I looked forward to being treated by her. She was exceptionally wonderful. I give them an A+.

WALTER A.: *NHL, High grade, 87 years old, male, disease-free two years*

Life One Year Before Diagnosis

I had a wonderful life. I had been very active in the town and the state. I even taught college. I knew what I wanted in life and I enjoyed life. I like to do a lot of things myself. I'm a hands-on person. Before my cancer, I was in good shape. (However), I had five bypasses 25 years ago, and not really have had a problem since then. I also have trouble in my left eye, which I still have. I get shots in my eye every two to three months. I take care of myself.

Diagnosis of NHL

I got a sore in my left cheek or nose. My wife, who was a doctor's assistant, knew all about these things. She referred me to a nose doctor and they took a biopsy and found cancer. When I was told I had cancer, I just accepted it. My wife and I both did. I take things as they're dealt to me. The guy up there *(God)* has been very good to me.

Treatment and Treatment Side Effects

I went to *(a hospital)* where they gave me radiation first in the left side of my sinus. I had chemo. It was supposed to be eight sessions, but I could only take seven. I had thoughts of committing suicide. I just almost wanted to die after about the sixth chemo treatment. It was a pain I've never experienced before. It was unbelievable. It's not a stabbing pain— it turns your head around, all in circles. For about three days your head is completely mixed up. It will last for a day and a half that you're in agony. Other than when I was really sick, I was working outside. I couldn't stay in the house and just sit down and read. That's not me. But the pain that I was getting in my head was just unbelievable. I also have problems in my left eye, which is not related to cancer. The shots I get in my eye every two to three months also sets off my brain and the pain in my nose and left jaw. I talked to several doctors at the hospital about my other medical problems too. They really don't know that much about what older people go through with this pain in your head.

Quality of Life During Treatment

Functioning

I'm hurting. *(Although it was difficult for me to)* go out to my garden, I took care of my yard. When I was lightheaded, which was a lot, I would hold onto the rake, or I would hold onto the bushes and rake with one hand, or hold my cane and rake with one hand. I push myself; I just didn't give in.

Relationships with Family, Friends, and Acquaintances

My doctor was very good, but it was my wife and my dog that got me through this. My wife is unbelievable. We've been married almost 65 years. I also have a collie *(dog)*. The collie would look at me and try to comfort me as much as possible.

DORIS R.: *NHL, disease stage not known, 88 years old, female, disease-free four years*

Life One Year Before Diagnosis

The year before I had the diagnosis wasn't too much different than several years before. From about the time my husband passed away, up until I was diagnosed, most every year seemed the same as the year before. I worked in a hospital for 20 years, and in the last four to five years, in a *(new floor for oncology patients)*. That was really the best place. I was an LPN *(licensed practical nurse)*. I did just about everything. We made beds, got patients up and dressed, gave them baths, did sterile dressings, and made colostomy bags *(external bags that collect feces for colon cancer patients who had part of their colon removed)* to stick on the patient.

I was lonesome sometimes because I'm far away from my family. Three of my daughters live in Michigan, and my other daughter lives in Utah. I'm way down here in Florida all by myself. I don't visit them and they don't visit me very often. They're all working and it's hard for them to get away all the time. I'm not one to try to interfere with anybody. I don't call them a lot, because I think maybe they would think I'm butting into their lives. My friends and I got together at exercise groups; that's been going on now for 18 years, with the same group of girls. We're almost just like sisters. I go shopping and go to church and do whatever I want to do. I just don't drive a car. *(Prior to being diagnosed with lymphoma, I had)* hypertension, low thyroid, and elevated cholesterol, and that was about it. All of that was controlled by medications. It really wasn't a problem. There was always a shortage of money. I get along, but I was always in debt. It wasn't too worrisome. I'm not too much of a worrywart actually.

Diagnosis of NHL

I got up one morning on Wednesday and looked in the mirror in the bathroom. I had a thick swelling in my neck. I had a feeling that it wasn't a benign thing—that it was something, not nothing. I started having difficulty swallowing and a little bit of difficulty breathing, a little breathless. The next day I went to my chiropractor. She said, "When you get home, promise me you'll call your doctor as soon as you get home." The doctor said, "Don't go home. I want you to go right straight to get a PET scan." I got the scan and then got a phone call from my doctor. He said he had the results and it was a mass. By that time I was having a little more trouble swallowing. My doctor sent me to an endocrinologist who thought that maybe it was a goiter. I said, "No, that's not a goiter. I know what a goiter is." He took a needle and drained some fluid out of this big thing. I got the report in two weeks. It came back benign. But the endocrinologist said that I'm having surgery to open this up, because he's still saying I had a goiter. They were going to take my thyroid out. After the surgery, the surgeon said, "You have lymphoma." I was relieved because they knew I didn't have a goiter. They left that big bulge on my neck. He said that he was going to send the cancer doctor over to see me. The cancer doctor said that they were going to use three different chemotherapeutic drugs on me. No surgery—"It wouldn't do any good. The lymphoma, it's all through your system."

Treatment and Treatment Side Effects

The doctor said, "There will be six treatments, one every three weeks." When I started to get the chemotherapy, that was pretty horrible. I was so sick. I didn't have much nausea, but it completely took away my appetite. Everything I ate tasted like wet cardboard. I think I lost 18 pounds, and I wasn't that big to begin with. It took about two years for me to get my appetite back. Along with the food tasting like wet cardboard, there was a terrible taste in my mouth. My mouth was so dry all the time I just drank water, drank water, drank water. It never seemed to help too much. I had night sweats so bad, mostly in the night, but in the daytime too. I'd wake up in the morning and my bed would be soaked. I didn't know if sweating was from the chemotherapy or the medications that I take. In addition, I was tired all the time and had pain in my stomach. The chemotherapy messed up my insides. I could sleep, but not for a long time. I'd go to bed at night and I'd sleep about

three hours. I'd wake up and maybe I could get back to sleep—
maybe not. It was the loss of appetite and the horrible taste in my
mouth *(that bothered me the most)*. The doctor said, "You're sick
and tired of being sick and tired."

Quality of Life During Treatment

Emotional State

I just felt sad. I guess you'd call it depressed, but I wasn't going to
blow my brains out. I always thought I'd get better. I had diabetes.
I had to have a hysterectomy. Everything that's happened to me
always got better. Now, I had the same feeling about this: "You're
going to get better someday. Just hang in there, kid."

Functioning

I didn't go to exercise for probably maybe eight months or so. I also
didn't go to church for six to eight months. *(Doing things was hard)*,
not only because I felt terrible, but I hardly had the desire or energy
to fix a meal.

Relationships with Family, Friends, and Acquaintances

My daughters were all still working. They called sometimes. They
never have been one to call me very often. Two of my daughters
came down to see me. One lives in Utah, and one lives in Michigan.
They stayed with me a couple of days. They were interested *(in coming to see me)*, but not living close by, they tend to forget *(to come and
visit)*. My friends called to see how I was doing. One of my friends
shopped for me and paid for my groceries with her own money.
I always think I should be the one doing for somebody else. My chiropractor said, "Let somebody do something for you. That makes
them feel good."

Religion

People at my church would pray for me. I was on the list they prayed for. I think it's got to have had something to do with my recovery. It felt good that people did pray for me, and I believe prayer has healing effects.

Satisfaction with Medical Care During Treatment

The cancer center where I went—those people were so nice. The nurse and the LPN were just so caring and upbeat. I think that's part of their duty.

AFTER TREATMENT AND THROUGH SURVIVORSHIP

FLNEWT: *NHL Mantle Cell Lymphoma, Stage IV, 67 years old, male, in-remission two years*

Late Treatment Side Effects

I have not had any long-term treatment effects.

Quality of Life after Treatment and Through Survivorship

Emotional State

I still do not have any concern of the cancer coming back, and if it does, we will deal with it. I am not sure that I will have the same attitude about beating the cancer if I relapse. One never knows just how a relapse will happen. My hope is that it does not.

Regaining and/or Changing One's Life

When I was first diagnosed, I was determined that my cancer would not limit my life. I had a sense that I would beat my Stage IV mantle cell lymphoma, although I knew it was incurable, but I am now in remission. While I continued to train for marathons and other running events, I had to physically reduce my training and cut my races back from full marathons to half marathons. I ran my first marathon just three months after starting treatment. I am planning to run enough marathons to reach the 100 half-marathon club.

Coping with Having Had Cancer

I've always had a positive attitude. I think that was a major factor in coping with the initial diagnosis. I used all the resources I could find to learn as much as I could about mantle cell lymphoma. I went to several websites including the Leukemia and Lymphoma Society and the Lymphoma Research Foundation, and read what I could about my disease. I also have a strong faith in God and knew my time had not yet come. I was determined to not only survive my diagnosis, but thrive because of it.

Overall Impact of Having Had Cancer

Negative and Positive Effects

I really never felt any negative effects from the cancer. I did cut back from running full marathons to running half marathons. That was due to dehydration, which could have been a part of my treatment. On the positive end, I've been able to encourage other people. I have one person at our church who is going through colon cancer. I arrived in the same room as her for chemo every so often, and I just kept encouraging her.

Greatest Concerns

I really don't have any major concerns. If the cancer comes back, I'll deal with it then. The state of the art is advancing so rapidly that I know there will be other options for me that could lead to a cure.

Advice

Reach out to friends, to family, and have a positive attitude. Those are the three most important things. It's also important to have certain long-term goals and also have some belief in a future afterlife.

LIL: *Large B Cell Lymphoma, disease stage not known, 69 years old, female, disease-free four years; Prior cancer: Uterine Leiomyosarcoma*

Long-Term Treatment Side Effects

I was taken by surprise by these long-term side effects, especially those that interfered with my physical activities. What I experience is tiredness and tremors. My memory is rocky. It takes me time to pull stuff up into the forebrain. My balance is really shot and the numbness in my toes is directly due to Vincristine *(one of the chemotherapy drugs)* and made me more prone to stumbling. So, I try to do balance exercises during the day. I practice restorative yoga and yin yoga, both of which are very helpful. They support relaxation and help me sleep. It's kind of like meditation. Probably more important is that I stay as physically active as possible to keep my body in shape, especially outdoors, with my friends and husband.

Quality of Life after Treatment and Through Survivorship

Emotional State

Doctors told me that I was not going to survive from having leiomyosarcoma, and that I would be lucky to get another number of months or years, and here I am. I can't be in the comfortable denial of death. I'm here, I'm enjoying this sunny day, and I know it could be taken away from me in any minute. I feel that every day, but I also experience a depth of appreciation for my life and the people I am close to.

Relationships with Family, Friends, and Acquaintances

My husband was absolutely fabulous and has been critically important all along for me. He was with me every step of the way. He is
my best friend, my coach. He is the son of Holocaust survivors. *(My
having cancer)* is not strange to him. He's very present-oriented and
I've learned so much from him about living in the present.

My friends have been great all the way through cancer treatment
and the aftermath. While I was in the hospital having the transplant,
my bike buddies were just great support. During chemo, they made
sure I got out, even if it was for a walk around the pond. But they
also got into mountain biking and really high-impact sports. I still
bike but I can't do *(mountain bike riding)*—I can't risk falling. So
I see less of those friends. I think without the cancer and the treatment I would be stronger at 69 years old than I am now. But I think
that I probably would not be any stronger emotionally or spiritu-
ally. I'm grateful for the experiences with having had cancer that
gave me that.

Sexual Life

I chose to learn and carry out years of my own internal, vaginal physical therapy so that I could stay sexually active in the way I wanted.
I think I have had a much more vibrant relationship with my husband than we would have if I decided this was too hard to do.

Regaining and/or Changing One's Life

I gave up teaching before I had the first cancer *(leiomyosarcoma)*.
I got the second edition of the book *(I wrote)* out in paperback,
and then I just stopped working professionally. I'm used to having
a purpose-driven life and working hard. I really want to find myself
engaged in a professional way again. I tutor English as a second lan-
guage and I run a support group for people with blood cancers, and

things of that nature, but not to a level of engagement as writing a book or teaching a class. It's just not happening for me right now.

I wanted the support of my friends in a way that was easy for them and me. CaringBridge, an online website, provided an easy way for patients who are facing serious illnesses to communicate with their friends and family. Basically, it is a blog where you can post what's happening to you to a closed group of people and they can reply. It eliminates repeated phone calls and text messages. CaringBridge was a huge help in coping with having had cancer, both during and after treatment.

After my treatment for lymphoma, one of the clients from the Breast and GYN Health Project and I decided that what we really needed was a lymphoma support group of our own, which would include both men and women with any kind of blood cancer. So, the Breast and GYN Health Project included us in their organization. After having NHL, I was called on mostly by the Breast and GYN Health Project to listen to the concerns of the newly diagnosed, answer their questions, steer them to wiser choices (*concerning their cancer treatment and resources*) when living in rural communities with limited resources.

It's been a big challenge post-treatment to adapt to a life (*focused on*) enjoying life. I'm going to do what I love to do, with the people I love. I would not want to give up the time that I spend with my grandniece and grandnephew. It is the high point of my week. That's my purpose for this year. I have a sense of the future now as I watch them grow. I've survived almost five years, and I'll probably survive for another decade or two.

Impact of Prior Cancer

When I was diagnosed with NHL, I already had my experience with leiomyosarcoma under my belt. With that first cancer, I was told it was an incurable sarcoma and that I had a maximum of three years to live, if I got radiation. I did the radiation. Ironically, that may well have led to NHL nine years later. I still have this cloud over my head.

I could have a recurrence of sarcoma at any time. I've had to learn to live with the knowledge that my future was uncertain. It really changed the way that I saw time and my life. I started living so much more in the present than I had before. I started a daily practice of gratitude. A close friend told me to "do something every day that keeps you in touch with the life force." For me, that is being in nature, being physically active, and time spent with the children.

Impact of Prior Non-Cancer Life Stresses on Coping with Having Had NHL

Before cancer, I had gone through a decade of hard psychological work on the pervasive sexual abuse in my childhood. Through that, I gained tools and insights that helped me cope with having cancer when it came. People who have similar histories of abuse can be destroyed by it. I was lucky and I was determined to own my own life. It was hard work.

Satisfaction with Medical Care after Treatment and Through Survivorship

I should have had a local oncologist now, but there was such a high turnover of docs, they were there for *(only)* a few months. And I had gotten such misinformation from generalists who didn't understand my particular cancers. So, for follow-up, I still take the two-day trip to the city to see my doctor at the cancer center.

Overall Impact of Having Had Cancer

Negative and Positive Effects

I have lost my sense of ambition. I don't have a focused drive. That could be a function of age; it could be a function of what I've been through, or something else altogether. There's been tremendous positives. I think that my relationship with my husband deepened. I feel so open to other people in ways that I wasn't necessarily before. I *(had been)* more caught up inside my own story, my own ambition, my own work. Now, I could spend time just sitting and talking with strangers, hiking in the forest. I ran into a young man and we had a nice conversation. That's not a friendship that's going to sustain me, but it's just one human being openheartedly in a conversation with another human being.

Advice

Get the best medical help you possibly can. Go to a major cancer center teaching hospital if at all possible. I don't think I would have survived without the experimental treatment. When I was diagnosed with the first cancer, my friend told me and my husband that we needed to build our own medical team. Seek out a medical center where they see hundreds of people with your diagnosis a year. You don't want an amateur. Finding the expert made all the difference for me. Seek out support from other cancer survivors. That's really tremendous because they know firsthand what it is you are going through. If you are lucky enough to have a dedicated support person, and I was, they need support and nurturing, too. They need time off. They need time with friends. They need to be listened to by someone else. And of course, they need appreciation.

Accepting help was really hard for me at first because I was used to being the helper, the one that got things done. I had to learn that when you let people help you, you're giving them a gift. They need a concrete way to express their love and concern. It's not a weakness to say, "I need your help."

ROY M.: *NHL, Grade 3, 70 years old, male, in remission one year*

Long-Term Treatment Side Effects

I had neuropathy in both feet. It doesn't affect balance. I think it was vincristine, but mine was not really that painful or disabling.

It probably limits my activities a little bit. I still have shortness of breath, more than I did before the transplant. It only affects my biking up a pretty steep hill. I have blood counts that are close to normal. I don't know if that's just aging or a long-term effect from chemo, but I am simply not as strong as I used to be. However, it doesn't affect daily living. The next thing is my memory. I don't know if it has anything to do with the chemotherapy or not, but I definitely have lost the ability that I once had to think really clearly and recall things. Other side effects I had during treatment pretty much went away.

Quality of Life after Treatment and Through Survivorship

Emotional State

I don't know if feeling better emotionally is totally due to cancer. Part of feeling emotionally better was our move to *(my current home)*. It was so much more stimulating *(than our prior home)*. I did support groups where people have said there's nothing good about cancer whatsoever. I think if you're going to deal with cancer effectively, somehow you'll have to deal with that anger. This anger that I had was simply no good. I finally understood that my anger was just self-destructive. That was true, not just for me, but to all those around me. But that can be hard to change without a pretty significant shot at feeling better after the treatments.

I think that as things went on, with lots of scans, my anxiety about my cancer coming back was reduced. Now I view a scan as just more information. I'm the type of person that feels that the more information I have, the better.

Regaining and/or Changing One's Life

What a patient wants is to get back to the life they had, if it was a good one. They have no patience for waiting x number of months.

I want to get back to the life I had now. It's very hard to control that feeling. I do have fatigue and shortness of breath. But for the cancer, I would probably still be lifeguarding and teaching swimming. Being a lifeguard is a bit of a stretch once we get past being 65 years old. I think the cancer affected my confidence, and it's just the type of thing you couldn't do anymore. There's too much risk in not being able to respond appropriately in an emergency. That was a loss. I don't think I had to give up anything entirely other than being a lifeguard, or markedly change anything I wanted to do, like bike riding. I love and am still able to bike ride. I am part of a biking team and we rode 36 miles. I cannot do that at the pace that I used to do it, but I'm not horrendously slower. That's why it's so important for cancer patients to set some goals. You have to push yourself.

Relationships with Family, Friends, and Acquaintances

Once I accepted some things that made me more tolerant, it probably improved the relationship with my wife and family. It certainly increases awareness on everybody's part of some things that just don't matter a whole lot, so let's not focus on those. My wife has always been incredibly caring, kind, and tolerant. The philosopher Henri Nouwen said, "A friend who can be silent with us in the moment of despair or confusion, who can stay with us in an hour of grief and bereavement, who can tolerate not knowing, not curing, not healing, and face with us a reality of our powerlessness, that is a friend who cares." *(posted on Permalink April 29, 2005)*. You ask yourself, "Where do we find those? Where do we find that kind of friend?" But you do. My wife is that friend.

I would like to have a more in-depth discussion with our son, about the chances that I won't survive. We had in place the appropriate wills, power of attorneys, health care, and so on. But *(at the medical center)* they were helpful in telling you how to talk to family members, particularly children, about these issues.

Communication

I think sometimes people just say, "You're a survivor. You've been around for five-plus years now, into your sixth year *(after you were diagnosed with having lymphoma)*. You've got to get over it." That's where support groups are so good. The captain of my biking team is on the executive board for a chapter of the Leukemia and Lymphoma Society. In their meeting, they talked about how hard it is for people that haven't gone through having had cancer themselves to know how to talk to cancer patients. One of the physicians on the board of this chapter said, "Yes, that would be a good topic for our next annual Leukemia and Lymphoma Conference. What are some ways that you can talk to a cancer patient? Part of it is being a good listener."

Coping with Having Had Cancer

What has helped so much, so obviously, is that the medical and science side has worked. I think the psychological side is always a problem. We have done tai chi *(type of exercise used to reduce stress by slow movements and deep breathing)* and it really helped to get back into that. I have done some work with meditation, and I think that has been helpful. Biking introduced me to a whole new group of friends, relationships, and activities. My wife does not bike, but we do all social events throughout the year. Gilda's Club has a bone marrow transplant group that meets once a month. I've gone to that. We definitely stay connected with them, but primarily our connection there is volunteering and obtaining financial support.

Coping Needs That Went Unmet

There isn't a whole lot of guidance for those of us who are at my age. You just don't find many therapists who know what the appropriate exercise limits are. I have found a fitness coach who is more attuned to working with cancer patients. Because so many people have cancer, this is something that can make their quality of life better.

Overall Impact of Having Had Cancer

Negative and Positive Effects

I expect that I will probably succumb to cancer eventually. This thing *(cancer)* sucks. There's no way I'm going to be positive. I've not been that optimistic a person during my lifetime. Having said that, I belong to an "Optimist Club," consisting of an optimistic group of people who meet every Tuesday.

Greatest Concerns

My concerns are about when I'm not here. You're walking through the valley of the shadow of death—getting things in place, wills, power of attorney, and all that stuff.

Advice

If you're living in a small community, and you're being treated at a community hospital, get a second opinion at a cancer center. Do it right upfront, because cancer is a very complex disease. When you have cancer, it's very helpful to move forward. Cancer makes you much more aware that dying is impending. If you're interested enough in exploring whatever it is you love, whether it's a new challenge or more physical *(activities)*, like biking, you are moving forward. It has had positive effects in my dealing with the disease. That's why every cancer patient I meet, I tell them to exercise, because I know you can recover from what seems to be some pretty dire physical problems. If you can't do any exercises, then walk barefoot on the grass around your house. I think nature can be very healing. There are a lot of support groups that can help with that. We have a large biking team where some of our members are very slow riders *(which include those who are older, or have physical limitations or disabilities)*. They have just as good a time *(as the rest of the bikers)*. It's not a race. In the spring we have a bike race, where you never leave anybody behind *(who are very slow riders)*. Someone has to ride slowly with that group, and that's fine. Also, identify the resources in your community. The Cancer Support Community, which includes Gilda's Club, is a good one. They have support groups. Sometimes the cancer centers have support groups. Last, hope is not necessarily just patients getting reports saying that you're in full remission. I don't think we win or beat cancer when you get that report. If you don't get those reports, don't let it strip the joy out of your life. That's how I think you deal with it in the best way.

STEVE: *NHL, Stage I, 70 years old, male, in remission one year*

Overall View of Survivorship

I don't think of myself as a "survivor" and don't wish to be called that. I have already relapsed four times. I have not survived the ordeal. I am living it in my mind and body every day. I hope this latest treatment doesn't fail me like the others.

Long-Term Treatment Side Effects

Today I suffer from severe peripheral neuropathy caused by all the cancer treatments. I'm in pain 24 hours a day. I'm in the pool in my condo every morning. Usually the pool gives me four to five hours where the pain is not real bad. There is really no help out there for someone like me. It is so frustrating not to be able to talk to someone else who's going through what I have or even find professionals who can help you. I've had every single possible drug these doctors could think of to deal with this peripheral neuropathy. There is nothing out there drug-wise that really deals with people who have peripheral neuropathy that comes from chemotherapy. I just don't have the energy anymore to do things. I used to love to go hiking and a steep hill was not a problem for me. I'm not going to be able to do that again because of the shortness of breath. That's not going away and it's something that's awful that I have to deal with. I'm just hoping that I can get to the point that I cannot relapse.

Quality of Life after Treatment and Through Survivorship

Activities

Because of my having ADHD *(Attention Deficit/Hyperactivity Disorder)*, I can't read a book—I can't concentrate. Most of my days right now, I come down to the club room in my building and put on music. On one of the TV stations, along with the music there are also inspirational sayings. It helps me stay hopeful and not afraid and believe that good things can happen.

Relationships with Family, Friends, and Acquaintances

The only connect I have is with my son. We have common interests in sports, in politics, and all types of things. We just like talking on the phone several times a week. I know he loves me. I just keep going because I don't want my son to feel the pain that I felt when my father died. We're basically best friends.

Coping with Having Had Cancer

I just always said, "You know something? You just got to hang in there and just keep on going and be hopeful that you can get something back in your life that you had before you got sick." You have fear, but I just never let the fear overtake me. I'm not willing to throw in the towel yet. I think that the main reason that I was able to cope was because I was in excellent physical condition when I started this whole thing. My whole life I have exercised seven days a week and I love it. I continued to exercise. When I was in that pool I felt like I was somewhat normal again. I felt good and I enjoyed it, and when I got done I felt better. The ability to do that tells me that there is hope, that everything hasn't been taken away from me. However, the pain and the problem with neuropathy concerns me more than really the cancer coming back right now. Now I know that, basically, if the cancer comes back, there's not much that I'm willing to do anymore.

My son is the reason I want to stay living right now. Talking over the phone with my son really helps. Knowing that he's doing well makes me feel like there's worth in my life still, and that maybe I can help him get through his daily routines sometimes. That's important to me.

Coping Needs That Went Unmet

The only people I want to talk to are the people who have gone through exactly what I have gone through, and what I'm going through now. That's where I feel I can learn something that's help-ful for me. I was forced to face the reality of the *(treatments)* that the oncologists were going to use. I just went ahead and did it. But my biggest regret is that I just didn't get enough information before *(being treated)*. I want information that will help me and give me a better understanding of how I can go forward with this thing. *(Not finding anything that worked to treat my pain)* doesn't keep me from looking every day to see if there is something new. But I'm realistic—there is nothing really out there. I have relapsed four times *(from treatments)* in the last five years. I can deal with the pain. It's awful, it's a horrible thing, but I live with it. I get through the day because my mind is clear. I just need to find a way to keep on going. I'm always looking for something that may give me some hope.

Satisfaction with Medical Care after Treatment and Through Survivorship

I know if my doctor comes across something that she thinks will help, she'll call me immediately, because I know that she is thinking about me. She wants to help me. She knows how I'm suffering. I realize that no doctor has enough time for me. They are so inundated just trying to do what they can for the people that they have to see every day.

I think that before oncologists give these horrible drugs to people, they have to explain to them exactly what the possible side effects are and how their life is going to be affected. I think that oncologists just give out the drugs without really having the patient understand what he/she is committing to. I wish that I would have had those options put forward to me by someone that I respected at that point in time, so I could make a decision and not just jump into it the way I did. So my point is, after you see the oncologist and the oncologist gives you his opinion of where you stand, these hospitals need to have people who you can talk to and ask hundreds of questions, and explain exactly what you are going to be going through and what you are going to be facing. Patients don't have enough information before we make these decisions. That is the biggest problem that we all face.

Overall Impact of Having Had Cancer

Negative Effects

Knowing what I know today, I would probably have done the orchiectomy *(removal of testicle),* but certainly would have gotten a second opinion and researched the available info before jumping into the surgery. Knowing what I know now and the ordeal I was going to face and the horrendous side effects I face now, I would have opted for watchful waiting and rolled the dice on what would happen next with the cancer.

Greatest Concerns

My biggest concern right now is the stiffening I have in my hands due to the neuropathy. Eventually, I won't be able to use my hands, and they're getting worse all the time. Right now, there is really nothing *(available to treat)* my problem.

Advice

You just don't jump into anything. You've got to get all information that's available and talk to as many people as possible before you make your decision. The oncologists are so busy—they don't have time for you. I never thought that *(NHL)* was going to kill me. I was always hopeful. You have fear, but I just never let the fear overtake me. You just have got to hang in there and just keep on going and be hopeful that you can get something back in your life that you had before you got sick.

RON: *NHL Burkitt's Lymphoma, Stage IV, 72 years old, male, disease-free four years*

Quality of Life after Treatment and Through Survivorship

Regaining One's Life

I said, "it's time that you get your body back." And from that point forward, I just started working out like I always worked out. I got myself back in shape, so that I could play tennis and go water skiing and snow skiing, and all the physical activities that I enjoy doing.

Satisfaction with Medical Care after Treatment and Through Survivorship

(The medical care) was wonderful. My oncologist is the sweetest person I could have gotten.

Overall Impact of Having Had Cancer

Positive and Negative Effects

I think the most positive and the most emotional thing were all the people that came forward to my aid. The other positive thing is I think it gave me the feeling that my body is really trying to do all it can do to keep me alive. There is no negative effect.

Greatest Concerns

The biggest issue for me, initially especially, was how do I continue to take care of my Mom and my aunt, when I can't even take care of myself? I do pay all their bills and make sure that they are comfortable at the assisted living home.

Advice

Keep yourself in the best shape you can. Stay away from drugs, stay away from smoking. If you're going to drink, drink alcoholic beverages in extreme moderation. I did all of that so that I could play tennis and water ski and snow ski and all the physical activities that I enjoy. That's the same advice that I was given and that the doctors said saved my life.

We just had a reunion with our high school friends this past weekend. I shared this story with them. When I give out the story, it's not a negative story. It's a story that says, "Hey, you can live through this. You just have to prepare yourself for it. So, if you want to put up a good fight against anything that comes your way, you got to be in shape for it."

KAYE C.: *NHL, disease stage not known, 74 years old, female, disease-free 2.5 years*

Quality of Life After Treatment and Through Survivorship

Emotional State

I think maybe I suffer from a bit of depression because I can't do what I think I'd like to do. I still have a very good life. I really do. I guess the basic is just I'm still alive. I'm pain free. Sometimes I worry about recurrence, whether it's stem cells or some other kind of cancer. Basically, under the circumstances, I think I'm doing quite well.

It was quite a fear *(that the cancer would come back)*, but the longer I've been cancer-free, the less frightened I am. But I've also made a decision. That is, that if it recurs, I'm not going to do anything about it. I don't want to go through this again. I don't want to put my family through it again. I'll just let nature take its course.

Regaining and/or Changing One's Life

I have not regained my strength—I just don't have the get-up-and-go. I think it's the physical activity that I miss a lot. I don't walk as far as I used to. I used to hike a lot in Arizona in the mountains. I don't do that anymore. I used to golf—I don't golf anymore. I only drive in neighborhoods that I'm familiar with. I don't feel comfortable driving outside my patch because I don't think my reflexes are what they used to be. I used to like to entertain a lot. We don't do that much anymore. I used to enjoy cooking. I don't find that enjoyable anymore. I used to be a big reader. Now I don't read anywhere near like I used to. I couldn't use a can opener. I just didn't have the strength in my hands and arms. I'm a little bit shaky. My taste buds have not fully returned. I eat because I'm hungry, but not because it tastes good. The doctors said that might not change.

I would like to gain some of my (strengths and activities that I like to do) back. I have been going to physical therapy. I've been doing my exercises. We were down in Tucson over the winter. I swam almost every day in the pool with exercises they gave me. When cooking, I do real easy things—a lot of frozen foods and things that don't take a lot of effort. Maybe it's the "new normal". (Activities I was able to continue doing were) playing bridge. I love to play bridge and playing with my grandkids. New activities were playing Words with Friends (an internet word game, similar to Scrabble), with friends from all over, from Arizona to California to Boston. I get a lot of enjoyment out of that, which I never did before. My kids gave me a Kindle and I read when I get up very early in the morning.

Sexual Life

(The treatment) did not affect my sexual life with my husband, but it has done more so now. My husband has been very understanding of it. We cuddle on the couch together, but intercourse hasn't been there for awhile.

Coping with Having Had Cancer

My family and my friends helped me *(cope with having had cancer)*. We have a large circle of friends in Minnesota and in Arizona. They've all been so helpful, so understanding, so encouraging. That's how I cope.

Overall Impact of Having Had Cancer

Negative and Positive Effects

My relationship with God has changed. I used to enjoy going to church. I got mad at God: "What did I do to deserve this?" I've been going to church more often now, but I still have a little bit of a chip on my shoulder. My inability or lack of ability to do a lot of things I used to do and enjoy doing, like driving and golfing—I'd like to get back to doing those things, but I'm not terribly encouraged. I take it one day at a time. Not a lot of positive effects because it has changed our lives.

Greatest Concerns

My biggest concern is my getting weaker and weaker. I think if I had more strength I could do more of the things I used to do with my family and friends. I just don't have this strength right now.

Advice

I wish other patients have the support group that I've had. I think you have to stick to a program, be it physical therapy or whatever. I think that's important. I think you've got to give it your best. Make the changes that make you feel better and do the best you can with what you've got. Just hang in there and be strong.

MARSHA JEAN LUNDMARK: *NHL, Stage I, 77 years old, female, disease-free 2.5 years*

Long-Term Treatment Side Effects

The radiation therapy destroyed one of the two salivary glands. My mouth is still dry, but I still have the other salivary gland. I can cope with it in the daytime, but at night, it wakes me up. You don't swallow as much in the night to refresh your mouth, and I still wake up with my throat completely dry and uncomfortable. Biotene is a gel that you can squeeze into your mouth and swish it all around and that can last for four hours. They also have a spray that you can spray in your mouth that makes it feel better. I only have to use Biotene at nighttime—in the daytime, there's no problem.

Quality of Life after Treatment and Through Survivorship

Emotional State

(When I go for the PET scan on a follow-up visit) you wonder if it's all clear *(no sign of lymphoma)* and if the next PET scan is going to be clear *(at the next follow-up visit)*. Basically, I just think that I will deal with that if it happens.

Regaining and/or Changing One's Life

I didn't have a whole lot of side effects, so I basically plugged along, maybe doing things slower, or maybe I'd have to skip weeding in the garden because I was too tired. But once the treatment was over, I went back to what I always did.

Coping with Having Had Cancer

I think God took all the fears from me—I didn't have them. I was very appreciative of the American Cancer Society, which bent over backwards to help me, as well as the Zonta Club, which provided the wig, and my doctors.

Overall Impact of Having Had Cancer

Positive Effects

(Having had cancer) really let me know how important I was to my family and that my grandson was so concerned.

Greatest Concerns

That I'd be able to live my life in my own home and not have to end up in a nursing home.

Advice

Have faith in God and He will bring you through it. Listen to your body. Nobody knows your body better that you do. If I hadn't kept looking at my throat, I would not have been so lucky.

ART B.: *NHL, Stage II, 80 years old, male, disease-free four years; Prior cancer: Acute Myeloid Leukemia (AML)*

Quality of Life after Treatment and Through Survivorship

Emotional State

I just don't worry about whether NHL is going to come back. There's a saying we use at Al-Anon: "If you are worrying about the future, you get anxious. If you worry about the past, you get a lot of resentments." I'd rather not be anxious or have resentments today. Today I'm doing OK. I live life as though I am normal. I don't keep it a secret that I had had these cancers *(NHL, AML)* because I know how much it helps when somebody comes to me and talks to me about this. There's nothing that I do different because I had had these cancers.

Other Non-NHL Cancer Problems

(In regard to my having AML before having NHL), the chemotherapy for AML caused short-term memory loss. I put something down, three minutes later I am looking for it. I have no idea where it is and when I left it. But half an hour from now, I will find it. The test showed that I did not have any dementia at all and no Alzheimer's, no other dementias. So now I don't get angry when I can't find something. I will say, "I know I will find it eventually."

I have severe sleep apnea. I was being awakened multiple times in an hour. They gave me a sleep apnea machine and that first night, I woke up so refreshed the next morning. It solved my problem with sleep apnea. I came close to fainting at a beach in Maine. No heart attack or other issues were diagnosed *(when I went to the emergency room)*. I was OK after a few hours. My cardiologist ordered a stress test that showed that my minor chest pains were not heart-related. I have assumed the fainting spell might have been due to dehydration. This has affected my home life because my wife now hovers.

Non-Medical Stresses

When I was diagnosed with follicular lymphoma, it was at the end of several deaths and illnesses. My mother died in 2006, my wife was diagnosed with breast cancer in 2006 and died in 2008, and my grandson died in 2009 due to drunk driving. Of those, the loss of my grandson was the hardest to accept. I was unaware that he had a drinking issue, so the shock was difficult to deal with.

Coping with Having Had Cancer

I have found that I have learned the difference between what I can do and what I can't do. I have no control over whether I have a disease, but I do have control over whether I find and accept treatment. My approach to treatment of my disease was an acceptance that treatment might not be available, or if available, not successful. I was surrounded by doctors and nurses and support people who provided whatever I needed to get well. While I did receive some negative news, I still recognized that the stats *(statistics)* they quoted were based on the past and was not a predictor of the future. This led me to avoid forecasting the worst and to live well today with whatever health I might have.

My Al-Anon community *(support group for family members and friends of alcoholics)* has been key to *(my coping)*. Al-Anon teaches me to do what I can and stop trying to do things I cannot. Those are kind of like my basic principles of living today. There's no question my eliminating isolation and being involved with others who have diseases similar to mine has been very helpful to me. *(During treatment)* there was one Wednesday night meeting where there were three other people who had had lymphoma who came to me after the meeting to *(talk)* about lymphoma. That was fantastic.

I remember there was a plane crash at Logan Airport. I had just gotten a job *(at Logan Airport)* that required me to travel. I had an internal discussion about whether I should give up the job. I didn't want to get in an airplane crash. Then I finally decided that I love my job. I developed this attitude of not worrying about death. *(After this)*, when I came to Al-Anon and they said, "Live in today; stop trying to change the past or forecast the future," that really was the basis for everything that has happened to me ever since.

Effect of Having a Prior Cancer on Survivor's Life

While I was being treated for AML *(prior cancer)*, I was doing what I could. I put together a 150-page book for this woman while I was being treated for AML. I was doing what I could. It gets you out of thinking "sick" and start thinking "I'm useful." Because I had survived leukemia five years earlier, I was well prepared to cope with having lymphoma. I was already in the Leukemia and Lymphoma Society (LLS) support group, already attending the LLS blood cancer conferences, and already still seeing my hematologist. I even had two years of grief support after my wife died of breast cancer. I didn't go into "Why me?" I was grateful that the lymphoma was treatable and that I had the support I needed.

Overall Impact of Having Had Cancer

Greatest Concerns

I think my greatest concern is wondering if this short-term memory is a thing that's growing worse *(due to AML treatment)*. I don't know if it's not going to get better or if it's going to stay the same. Losing my mind is probably the biggest fear I have.

Advice

The first thing is get a second opinion. Whatever the doctor says, get a different doctor to look at you. If you get the same answers, then you know you're in the right course. If you get a different answer, get a third opinion so you get a consensus. Second, don't worry about the future. You might not have one. Do things today that you want done or can do.

JUDY M.: *NHL, Stage II, 80 years old, female, disease-free three years*

Quality of Life after Treatment and Through Survivorship

Emotional State

I don't fear a recurrence. I figure if I have a recurrence of cancer of any kind, just go in there and get it taken care of. If the doctors can help, they will. If they can't, we'll just have to see what happens. I try to keep a positive attitude.

I did get depressed when we first moved down here because not only was I still recovering from all this stuff, but I also had my problem with my leg and knee. I was in the hospital for a few days while they were trying to figure out if it was cellulitis.

Regaining and/or Changing One's Life

I was tired for a long time. I would sit and nap in my chair in the afternoon. It was just such a gradual thing just to get over it, to get your strength back. I pretty much had kept up doing all the things I had been doing before *(I had cancer)* and I had to keep up rehab all through this too. After the chemo was done, I had my other knee replaced, and rehab after that. I was doing all these things. Sometimes I was tired and I didn't do *(rehab exercises)*, but other times, I was doing OK. It took probably six months to get my strength back, probably half due to my knee. The knee replacement was probably good because it was a distraction *(from having cancer)*. It also kept me physically doing something.

Relationships with Family, Friends, and Acquaintances

It's hard leaving a lot of people *(when you move)*, but as we've gotten older, we've seen a lot of neighbors move to other places and a lot of them die in nursing homes. There's nobody around anymore. Our neighborhood had not been a friendly neighborhood and we didn't get together much. We were involved in the church and then in work, and those were the only two places we had friends from. It just got to the point where we had to go somewhere else. We moved into *(our new home in Virginia)* and didn't know anybody. There was nobody around. I was rather depressed for a while, but then I started meeting people and joined a church. It's all been good.

Coping with Having Had Cancer

The experiences I had when I was a volunteer at the American Cancer Society probably helped me a lot because I knew a lot about cancer, although not recent stuff *(as I had left ACS in the 1990's)*. Religion also helped me. We've always been churchgoers. My husband and I belonged to the church choir for 50 years and have done everything else in the church you could think of. There's a strength that you receive from that.

Satisfaction with Medical Care after Treatment and Through Survivorship

When we moved down to Virginia, I had to go to a new oncologist, and he was wonderful. He said, "If any of this cancer doesn't show up again, I consider you cured." He retired after I was here for six months. Now I'm going to another oncologist whose specialty is lymphoma, and he's good.

Overall Impact of Having Had Cancer

Negative and Positive Effects

I don't think there was a negative impact of having had cancer. Positive—yes. I probably have more empathy now. For people who are not well, whether it's cancer or anything else that I also had, I realized that I felt that way too.

Greatest Concerns

(My greatest concern is) staying as healthy as I can and having my husband stay as healthy as he can, so we can enjoy this new life which we've created down here *(new home in Virginia)*.

Advice

Stay positive; look on the positive side of it: "I'm going to beat this thing." If something isn't feeling good, feeling right, get it checked out. I think it's important that older ones especially should keep busy and do as much they can. That's what helped us *(getting through my having had cancer)*, and will help you going forward as you get older.

PERL: *NHL, Stage IIIA, 81 years old, male, in remission 2.5 years*

Long-Term Treatment Side Effects

The doctor told me, "You're not going to feel up to par for probably about a year, because it takes a body that long to get rid of the chemotherapy. You're in remission, but I can't tell you that you're cured, because this cancer or any cancer could come back anytime. Let's think positive."

Quality of Life after Treatment and Through Survivorship

Regaining and/or Changing One's Life

I used to do about an hour workout every day. *(At first, after chemotherapy ended)* I did the hour, but I couldn't do what I used to do before I was diagnosed with cancer. I was very frustrated. I did get back to a normal life, but it took me over a year to get my strength back. Now I'm back to riding my Harley *(motorcycle)* and doing everything I can.

Other Non-Cancer Medical Problems

When I had my CT scan, they found out that I had two aneurysms besides the cancer. One of them is at the point where it had to be operated on because it was an abdominal aneurysm. The doctor said, "If that thing bursts, you could bleed to death." I said, "I'm not going to worry about that until we take care of the cancer first." When I was in remission and I had *(the aneurysm)* repaired, that hurt me more than the cancer did. The pain was horrendous from that repair and that stuck with me for probably two or three weeks.

Coping with Having Had Cancer

The things that helped me most were keeping a positive attitude, keeping my body in shape as much as I could by continuing to go to the YMCA, my religion, and my wife. A lot of people don't believe there's power in prayer, but I'm a real believer in that. I'm more of a believer now because I'm sure God helped as much as my positive attitude. One of the biggest things *(that helped me cope)* is my wife who helped me so much. If she sees me down, she picks me right up again. I pray every day that our loving relationship goes on for many years.

Overall Impact of Having Had Cancer

Positive Effect

The cancer has not really changed my life, but it made me thankful for at least what I have now. The health I have and my age, 81 years old, and I'm doing what I want to do. That has given me a continued attitude that I love life and hopefully I can continue having life for a long time.

Greatest Concerns

As I get older, I don't want to have another traumatic thing like a heart attack. I shouldn't worry about that because if it happens, it happens. I'm just going to try to keep it out of my mind, although I do think about that stuff now and then.

Advice

I know cancer scares you. That word itself is a terrible scare. But I would say keep as much of a positive attitude as you can, try to do your normal daily living, and keep your body in shape as much as you can. If you keep your body in shape, it's easier to fight the cancer. Whether you're religious or not, do some praying, but God helps you no matter what. He helps everybody.

BARBARA G.: *NHL, Stage IV, Grade 1–2, 85 years old, female, in remission two years*

Quality of Life after Treatment and Through Survivorship

Regaining and/or Changing One's Life

Because I had no bad side effects I was able to continue with most of the activities I had been involved in *(before I had lymphoma)*. The only thing that I have given up because of the lymphoma is bicycle riding, and I miss that. I continued going to exercise classes, the two book groups, the writing group and courses in the Learning in Retirement program. My plate is very full.

Emotional State

I am relaxed about getting the CT scans every year because it's been good for so long. I expect everything is going to be fine, so I don't worry about it. It's not something that's always on my mind, but nonetheless it's there. I realized I am very, very fortunate and my health otherwise is good. And, it's good despite the cancer right now.

Other Non-Medical Stresses

My older daughter, who lives with me, has been a recovering alcoholic for four to five years. Things have not always gone well for her. She was in a very stressful job which she finally quit and now is looking for another job and that's stressful for her, and for me as well.

Overall Impact of Having Had Cancer

Greatest Concerns

My daughter is my greatest concern. However, she is a recovering alcoholic and that pleases me. That's the biggest stress that I have.

Advice

Find someone that you can trust to be your caregiver, like your doctor. I think if you have faith in what he or she tells you, that's very helpful. My primary care doctor was the one that became concerned about my blood count. I was attributing my being tired to my age and would not have done anything about trying to find out why I was lethargic. Because of my primary care doctor, I was diagnosed and successfully treated. So, I think that health care that you are able to hook into is very important.

I think it's also important that you are able to share the fact that you are being treated for cancer. I know that some people try to hide the health problems that they have. I don't think that's a healthy thing to do. I think friends or family can be most helpful when they know what it is you are going through and so I would be open and suggest people be open about that.

WALTER A.: *NHL, High grade, 87 years old, male, disease-free two years*

Long-Term Treatment Side Effects

It has been two and a half or three years since I had cancer, and you'd think by now it would be OK. But every once in a while, maybe every third or fourth day, I would get this recurring pain. It goes in peaks. It goes right up to your nose and into your head and branches over to your eye. I just have to lie down for maybe five minutes now, and then it goes away. You never lose it—it's always with you. There's a spray you can use for your nose and you can take narcotics. My doctor says to me, "You're 87 years old. Why don't you take narcotics? It will make you feel better." It was something that was drilled into me, "Don't take narcotics, you'll get a habit." My granddaughter says, "Maybe you ought to try marijuana." But *(my hospital)* is not set up for marijuana.

Quality of Life after Treatment and Through Survivorship

Emotional State

I've had a great life. I tell everybody I'm the luckiest guy in the world. I don't have a million dollars in the bank and I didn't win the lotto. I just accepted having had cancer. Whatever God is going to tell me and give me, that's it. He gave me a hell of a good life. When I was younger, I was active in my town. But as I got older, when I hit my 80s, I just relaxed and enjoyed my life. But now I can't go up to the roof of my house. I've lost all of my friends—they passed away. I'm starting to be like a zombie.

Relationships with Family, Friends, and Acquaintances

My wife and I do everything together. If it wasn't for her, I wouldn't be alive. I love my son and grandchildren and I have a baby great-grandson who we love and thank God for. One of the biggest things that my wife and I look forward to is seeing pictures of my great-grandson and grandchildren.

I'm the type of person that doesn't want to bother other people. I was always very independent. My nephews knew when I was going through chemo, so they came to my home to cut my grass and plow the snow. My son came over a couple of times, but he lives an hour away, has three kids, and is very busy in his job. My daughter is busy too. My sister was very good to us. My brother-in-law just took my wife to the doctor now. It's a close family and we love each other to death. But we are just independent.

Other Non-Cancer Medical Problems and Stresses

Due to my heart problems I have a problem breathing; I'm gasping for breath. I am scheduled for an operation *(in a month)*, which is a long way off. I can't do the things I want to do. That's for sure.

We're lucky we had money, but the money is dwindling now. We figured that we have a house that's worth between five hundred to six hundred thousand dollars that we're going to have to do something with. We can only stay here another three years and then my money runs out.

Coping with Having Had Cancer

My wife was always behind me, who helped me cope, as well as my dog. There are a lot of people who can't quite accept they have cancer, and break down. I don't look behind me too much. What's happened in the past, I can't change. What's in front of me, I can change. I always felt that way. If I was not a fighter, I wouldn't be here.

What I really wanted to do and *(another hospital)* can't do *(because of the cost)* is talk to other people that have cancer. They are going through the same thing I am. Everything is addressed for those 60 years old at the other hospital. Nobody wants to write about older people. But we're still alive. We still have feelings. Maybe somebody can pick up this book *(Older Survivors of Cancer)* and say, "I'm normal. The book is written for people like me."

Satisfaction with Medical Care after Treatment and Through Survivorship

Just three years ago, cancer doctors thought that because you're older they let you off *(don't treat you)*. There was less sensitivity and knowledge about patients who were getting increasingly older. The doctors looked at you and said, "You're 85 years old. You're lucky to be alive." They don't do that anymore. I noticed that their attitude is completely different. *(My hospital)* has a group of cancer doctors and they have meetings all the time, and discuss with other doctors at other hospitals what's going on. The doctors are much more understanding. Communication is very good between the doctors and their cancer patients. That's probably true for many of the hospitals, but maybe not all.

Overall Impact of Having Had Cancer

Positive Effects

I would love to talk to other people that have cancer. Maybe try to cheer them up a little.

Greatest Concerns

Probably 99% of my worrying right now is taking care of my wife. In addition, another great concern is my problem with breathing. I'm on oxygen right now. It helps me, but I still have 50% discomfort all the time. I know the pain from cancer is going to go away, but not the problem with breathing.

Advice

I think communication is the biggest factor. I think people would like to share with other cancer people and say, "I'm not the only one that has it." I'm all by myself on an island. I think that if people could get together and no matter what cancers you have, we just talk it over. I think people would feel a lot better. I know when I talk to people with cancer, I feel a lot better. We understand each other. I think we grasp the situation a lot easier *(than those who haven't had cancer)*.

DORIS R.: *NHL, disease stage not known, 88 years old, female, disease-free four years*

Long-Term Treatment Side Effects

I think after the chemo was finished I did have some problems. I've still got AFib *(atrial fibrillation of the heart)*. I'm pretty sure the chemotherapy was the beginning of that. I have stomach trouble, and I have at times chronic diarrhea ever since I had the chemotherapy. I've been trying to control it, but I still have loose stools every two to three weeks. I've also got some neuropathy in my fingertips and feet. My feet feel like I'm walking on wet sand in cardboard boots.

Quality of Life after Treatment and Through Survivorship

Functioning

(*Because of the neuropathy in my feet*) my feet stay uncomfortable all the time. I used to be quite a walker—I loved to walk. Now, I might be able to walk a short city block. That would be about it. When I go to the grocery store, I use their grocery cart. By holding onto the grocery cart, that helps a lot when walking in the store. I'm a little off-balanced too. Next thing I'll be needing is a walker, and I hate the thought of that. Of course, you'd expect people of my age wouldn't do much walking anyway.

Emotional State

It doesn't take too much to make me happy. It doesn't take too much to make me cry a little bit. I get teary-eyed.

Relationships with Family, Friends, and Acquaintances

I'm lucky if somebody calls me once a month. I keep telling my kids now, "Why don't you call me?" I could be lying dead in this house for three or four days before anybody knows it, because nobody calls me. But I do call my brother and we get along really well. We always make each other laugh. My oldest daughter and her family I think are in a better position to come and visit now. They come every year in the winter time, for a week or so. It's nice to have them come. They always send me boxes of meat for special occasions, like Mother's Day, my birthday, and Christmas. I used to wonder when my kids were small and I was so overwhelmed, I'd be blessed if all were grown and were out of here. Now, I wish them back.

I have one good friend—my best friend. There were seven or eight of my friends who sat together in church. Now they are all gone—they either moved out of the area or just don't come anymore. I sit next to myself. I still don't have the energy to fix a meal. You eat alone. It's hard to eat alone all the time. Now I bring my supper plate in and eat in front of the television. That helps—I don't feel so lost.

Coping with Having Had Cancer

I miss church if we don't go. That really seems to be a part of my life. People would hear I was sick and they prayed for me. Even the guy that mows my lawn. One day when I opened the door and gave him his check for mowing my lawn, he said that he put me on the prayer chain *(group of people who pray together)* at his church. That felt really, really good. There are times in my life when I was kind of having a low spot. I could tell that somebody had prayed for me. I don't know how to explain how it felt, but I could tell that years ago when I was having trouble with some problems, and I can't remember what they were now, but I had this definite feeling that somebody prayed for me.

Overall Impact of Having Had Cancer

Negative Effect

The only *(negative effect that)* I can think of was that it seemed like time wasted. I could have been doing something else, something useful, and I keep thinking, even today, that God isn't going to take me because He's got at least one more thing that I'm supposed to do. "You keep me, Lord, because I know you got more things for me to do, and I don't know what it is yet, but I'm waiting."

Greatest Concerns

My greatest concern now is encroaching disabilities with old age.

Advice

There's a better day ahead. Don't give up until you can't do it anymore. Ask God to protect you and show you the way. You'll be all right. Listen to the doctor—pay attention. Take somebody with you when you go to the doctor—somebody who knows what the doctor is talking about.

Chapter 4

Older Survivors of Lung Cancer

As 228,820 lung cancer patients were diagnosed in 2018, lung cancer became the second largest type of cancer when compared to all other types of cancer in the United States. The percentage of cancer patients who were diagnosed as having lung cancer increases with age: 65–74 years old: 65.9%; 75-84 years old: 73.4%; 85 years old and older: 90.3% (National Cancer Institute, SEER Cancer Stat Facts). The rate of survival of five years or more is low, as it is approximately one-fifth (20.5%) of lung cancer patients. While the percentage is low, 20.5% survival translates into 46,908 lung cancer survivors, which is a significant and encouraging number of survivors when compared to prior decades when the five-year survival rate was only 5%. Those who were treated at an earlier disease stage (Stages I and II), often, but not always, have an easier treatment compared to those with more advanced disease (Stages III and IV). For this reason, lung cancer survivors' disease stage is given at the beginning of each participant's story.

The major issues that older lung cancer survivors experience that affect their ability to cope with having had cancer include physical and mental problems, the quality of their relationships with family and friends, the number of medical problems they have in addition to lung cancer, the role of religion in their lives, and the number of losses of important people in their lives, such as family members and close friends. A large study was done of the quality of life of older cancer patients who had any of nine different cancers, four of which are part of this book (NHL, bladder, colorectal, and lung cancer).

Two years after diagnosis, a significant decrease was found in older lung and colorectal cancer patients' mental and physical health (Reeve et al. 2009). Older lung cancer patients' decline in all of these areas was the worst when compared to patients with any of the other eight cancer diagnoses.

The list of issues mentioned above, which affected their being able to regain their lives after the end of treatment, are common to patients with *any* of the cancer diagnoses, not just lung cancer. What is unfortunately unique to lung cancer patients is the *stigma* placed on them by others for getting this disease. "They chose to smoke—it's patients' own fault that they got lung cancer." This kind of response from others can ruin their relationships and has been found to be significantly related to patients' psychological distress and overall quality of life (Chambers et al. 2015).

Reading this chapter you will see how the different participants experienced and coped with having lung cancer. For example, in this book, one participant talked about her son and two of her cousins who had died, in addition to her chronic back pain, which limited her standing and walking. This was in addition to having had broken ribs, pneumonia, the flu, and a broken foot. Across the board of all cancer diagnoses, as older cancer survivors age, it is not uncommon that the number and/or severity of medical problems increases, along with an increasing loss of those who were loved and cared about. Just having one of these problems can be sufficient to be a major problem in coping as they age. Having multiple major non-cancer problems becomes overwhelming. In one study of lung cancer patients, having just two non-cancer medical problems was the "tipping point" for experiencing the greatest impairment in functioning (Lowery et al. 2014). It's not surprising that older cancer survivors need to cope with more than just having had cancer.

INTO AND THROUGH TREATMENT

KATHY V.: *Lung Cancer, Stage IB, 68 years old, female, disease-free one year*

Life One Year Before Diagnosis

The year prior to my diagnosis was *(spent)** dealing with *(my husband)* and then losing him and then trying to figure out who I was, because I wasn't a wife anymore. I had all the issues that come with being alone, when you've lived with someone for 40 years.

During my husband's illness and death, I had been taking medications for anxiety, prescribed by my family doctor. She had been monitoring me this whole time. She's the only doctor that checks up on my emotional needs. I might add that I tend to be positive and upbeat at my medical appointments, which might lead the medical personnel to assume I'm fine—not necessarily something that should be assumed.

Diagnosis of Lung Cancer

At the time of being diagnosed with transient global amnesia *(a once-in-a-lifetime event causing loss of memory)*, a CT scan and MRI were done. The pulmonologist reviewed my scans and a nodule on my lung was detected. It was an incidental finding. The pulmonologist came in and said, "There's something ugly on your lung, only Stage I or II." *(I said)* "I can't deal with this because I just lost my husband." *(The pulmonologist)* took my hands in his and said, "I'm going to take care of you. You don't have to worry, because I'm going to take care of you."

---

* *Italicized (slanted) typing is used in parentheses when quoting participants to complete their sentences, in order to make the quotes clearer.*

(My medical oncologist) was very kind. He hugged me and we talked about *(my husband)* too. He said "Stage I with lung cancer is not the same as Stage I with other cancers. There's a higher probability of recurrence. There's a 40% or more chance that it will recur at Stage I." I came home and I just sat in the house and I realized that depressed me. It was the first time I had a feeling about my diagnosis. Then I realized that's actually a good thing because it meant I wanted to live. I did not have this "Oh my God" feeling that people talk about when they hear the words "You have cancer." I didn't hear that because I was still so numb from losing *(my husband)* that it was kind of like, "OK, I'll deal with it." I didn't go berserk or crazy. When I would get that concerned I just kind of went, "Well, I'll do whatever I have to."

Treatment and Treatment Side Effects

I had surgery and I was staged at IB. *(no further treatment was done after surgery)*. Breathing was a little more labored.

Quality of Life During Treatment

Emotional State

Sometimes people don't want to talk about it because they think they're going to upset you. To me, I get upset myself; it's not coming from other people.

Relationship with Family, Friends, and Acquaintances

Both of my sisters are nurses. My older sister called every weekend. I formed a relationship with my brother, who also wanted to help, and he was here when I needed him. And I have good friends here. They bring meals over. There were so many people who bent over backwards for us.

Communication

One of the things that matter most is how people say, "How are you?" when they don't want to know. People always say that and I just say "I'm great" but people would say to me right after they found that I had Stage I that it didn't sound as terrible. This one woman came up to me and said "You must be so happy." I looked at her and what I wanted to say was, "I still have cancer." *(Others asked):* "Did you smoke?" Lung cancer has a stigma to it. It doesn't matter whether I smoke. I have it and accepting that they're not going to give me sympathy or not sympathy. I haven't met many people like that. I know what <u>not</u> to say to people who have cancer: "Give me a call if you need anything." You say something specific: "Which day do you want me this week to make dinner for you, because I'd love to do it."

Coping with Having Cancer

I don't know how I coped. I have faith. I don't think that my faith is as deep as my husband's. I just kept myself busy. That's how I coped, I think.

Satisfaction with Medical Care During Treatment

Starting with the pulmonologist, he was wonderful, compassionate, and filled me with comfort. I couldn't ask for more from him. The thoracic surgeon I saw next, and he came in the room and he said he had been backed up because he had some emergency at the hospital so my appointment was delayed. He acted like I was the only person on his schedule. He listened. With him I felt that I was in very capable hands. He sat back in the chair next to us, not at the desk, and explained everything with pictures and explained what he was going to do and just gave me all the time we needed. That's really important.

ISABELLA: *Lung Cancer, Stage IV, 70 years old, female, in remission 1.5 years*

Life One Year Before Diagnosis

I retired from my job, because we had to if at the end of the year you were 65. I continued to work for them per diem until November of 2012 when I had both my knees replaced. Then I recovered for three or four months and went back to work, again part-time, two or three days a week, and loved it.

Diagnosis of Lung Cancer

I talked to the doctors. They ordered an X-ray and it was a big mass and in a span of a day I lost not only my health, but my job, which wasn't just a job, it was a career that had spanned since youth. Part of that was because it was felt at the time that I was a chemo emergency, that I had so much disease that they really needed to start chemo right away.

The beginning was extremely traumatic, because everything changed. I went from being a perfectly happy, capable, semi-retired person loving my work, to a sad person. The bottom line is I never went back to work. It took me awhile to adjust to being retired, but then after awhile I decided I liked it.

Treatment and Treatment Side Effects

I got a phone call from my oncologist who said, "I have good news: You're EGFR-positive, and there's a drug for it." *(Tarceva)*. I started Tarceva *(which had)* lots of side effects. I really didn't have horrid side effects. I got eight rounds of heavy-duty chemo, during which time I would say I was largely zombified *(turned into a zombie)*. I had virtually no energy, which then got worse and worse as the chemo continued. That was a very quiet period, quiet misery, during which time I did little, if anything. I had nausea until they switched meds, and then that got better, continuous diarrhea that makes you have to go, skin rashes that make you look like a teen-ager with acne, hair growing in various places you don't want it to grow, and not growing in places that you do want it to grow. I don't care. I mean if hair was growing where it shouldn't, I got rid of it. If it wasn't growing as it should, I covered it. I can't cope with 5,000 problems—I just have to manage. It's not to say that I never had a moment where it wasn't a pain in the ass, but things like that didn't bother me—I couldn't care less.

Quality of Life During Treatment

Emotional State

"Devastation" would be a good word.

Relationships with Family, Friends, and Acquaintances

I have two special needs adult kids that were with me *(along with my grandbaby)*. I was devastated that they were going to have to fig-ure out how to live on their own *(without me)*. That I would never see this baby *(my granddaughter, Sophie)* grow up. Sophie is a big responsibility for me because basically I'm raising her. Fortunately, she's just delicious. She is the light of my life. I think most of my friends didn't know what to do, but my closest friend would have done anything and she offered. I didn't have her do a lot but she did get copies of all the bits of DNR *(Do Not Resuscitate order)* paper to make all the hard decisions.

Various people offered to come to chemo and other things, when I discovered that these people were more trouble *(than expected)*. If you send some to the pharmacy they would get lost, or they would be a problem and they would get agitated. Then they weren't com-fortable sitting and doing nothing which is basically what I needed them to do. I really didn't need much. I just sat there and played on my tablet, waiting until it was over. It wasn't a big deal. One nurse was lovely. The most important thing for me was to have someone to talk to. They don't really know what to do and what to say. Most of them didn't do anything awful, thank goodness, or even say anything awful. At first I didn't tell everybody. I didn't keep it a secret kind of thing but I didn't put it out on Facebook. I wasn't sure I really wanted certain people to know, possibly because I intuited they wouldn't handle it well and say something insensitive, like "You need to deal with it." I think I kind of limited myself to people who I felt would handle it well. I would say my work colleagues were the least helpful. They all said, "That's terrible," then disappeared with nary a phone call.

Religion

Religion was a help only because my rabbi was such a help. At first it was really basically only the rabbi. I knew I could trust him and I knew I liked him. I knew what a mensch *(upstanding person)* he was. He helped with getting me to make final plans for my funeral. What they *(Jewish congregation)* do is they assign three people to you, who you get to approve, and those three people keep checking in on you. I had one who checked in on email, one who checked in on phone and one was texting. After my son had his accident and I was still not well, *(members of the congregation)* had weeks of meals delivered and they were very wonderful. This congregation is very unusual. It's just joyful.

Satisfaction with Medical Care During Treatment

I wasn't *(satisfied with the medical care)*. Some intern referred me to Pulmonary. It took them forever to get an appointment, like a week. Then they couldn't get a CAT scan and a schedule, then they thought I should see a surgeon. I was waiting for weeks and then

I got mad. I picked up the phone and called a girlfriend, who was an oncologist. By the time I got parked and in her office, the chart was up, the X-rays were up. She looked at everything. She sat down, immediately gave me the meds I needed for chemo, set up a bunch of biopsies. She took over and *(that)* was fine. I really didn't expect something spectacular from them, to fall down dead because I was a colleague. But I did expect them to be professional and do their jobs.

SUSAN OS: *Lung Cancer, Stage IIIA, 71 years old, female, disease-free one year*

Life One Year Before Diagnosis

Everything was good.

Diagnosis of Lung Cancer

The first sign I had was that I was coughing. *(After seeing the internist, and antibiotics didn't work,)* I went to see a pulmonologist. When I didn't respond to that second course of antibiotics, he gave me a chest X-ray and then I was diagnosed with lung cancer.

Treatment

I had four rounds of chemotherapy, lobectomy of the left lung, and 30 rounds of radiation.

Quality of Life During Treatment

Relationship with Family, Friends, and Acquaintances

My husband is wonderful to me. He makes dinner every night. He's very caring. I got to see wonderful qualities that he didn't show before. I used to do so much work around the house and now I do very little. I used to cook all the dinners. I don't do that anymore.

He does it. It probably made me better. I'm lucky. I'm close with my brother. I hear from him at least three, four times a week. I think it might be a little more now *(than before having cancer)*. My husband's daughter and husband live a couple of blocks away from us. Not once have they ever inquired how I am or in any way offered any kind of sympathy. When I was in the hospital having surgery, they came, stood at my bed. I have some friends who were very supportive. They called and asked me how I'm doing, which was nice.

Satisfaction with Medical Care During Treatment

The medical care I got at *(the cancer center)* gets an A+. I put myself in the hands of experts. I have total confidence in my surgeon. He is the master of the scalpel, because I didn't have a single moment of pain. I got all the help I needed. I thought every person in that hospital, from the lowest to the highest, from the people that check you in, to the people that take your blood, everybody was great, *(except for the radiologist)*. When I had gone through 28 out of the 30 radiation sessions, I said *(to the radiologist)*, "What's my prognosis?" He said, "You're going to die." I didn't understand it because my surgeon told me that I'm cancer-free.

CHERYL L.: *Lung Cancer, Stage I, 72 years old, female, disease-free three years; Prior cancer: Multiple Myeloma*

Life One Year Before Diagnosis

At the Lymphoma and Leukemia Society, I am what is called the "first connection." If somebody is newly diagnosed with multiple myeloma *(prior cancer before being diagnosed with lung cancer)*, and they have nowhere to turn, they could call the Lymphoma and Leukemia Society (LLS). LLS then asked me to be a "mentor" to those patients, which involves meeting with them on a one-to-one basis, providing them with friendship, caring, and information. I was pretty happy doing that and have continued to be the "first connection" to patients to this day. We had a Cancer Support Community in Sarasota, which I participated as a volunteer for 11 years *(prior to having lung cancer)*. At the Jewish Family and Children's Services, I would go to their meetings to "spread the hope," telling people how long I've been in remission *(from prior cancer, multiple myeloma)*. That's the first thing they love to hear. While I was at the Wellness Community I developed a Speaker's Bureau, which involved finding patients who were in remission or disease-free to tell their stories about their having had cancer. This has continued to this day. In addition, I became involved in the public speaking end of the Wellness Community. The outreach coordinator would take me to whatever speaking engagements she had, which included both hospitals and nursing homes.

I decided to join an Improv class *(art of acting and improvising, without any prior experience)* at the Florida studio theater. I was on my last breath practically. At the end, we did a performance—I was always full of laughter. *(During this time,)* I was in constant pain from my back. I was not able to walk more than 100 feet before I had to sit down. That derailed a lot of my activities. I would also get very tired. I *(also)* had tooth problems. You know if you ever had tooth problems, they can really hurt and it kills your life.

Diagnosis of Lung Cancer

At the time that I found about lung cancer, I was struggling with horrible back pain. It has been going on for years, but I had ways to make it better: acupuncture, non-narcotic drugs for arthritis, physical therapy. Nothing worked. Went to my spinal surgeon, *(Dr. G,)* who said: "I see a spot on your lungs. I would like for you to immediately tell your oncologist to have a good close look at it." I did and it truly was cancer of the left lung, and it was Stage I. I also had cancer in my pelvis and in my brain.

Treatment and Treatment Side Effects

The doctor at (*the cancer center*) simply went into my lung and removed the lower left lobe. The most important thing I had to overcome was breathing. That was very tough. I get out of breath quickly. The miracle about this little thing that happened is that if *(Dr. G)* had not been so sharp enough to see what he saw by accident, I would never have known.

Quality of Life During Treatment

Emotional State

One thing needs to be sure—where there is life, there is hope. That's all I had to keep feeling and I felt it. Having had multiple myeloma *(prior cancer)*, my husband and I were a little more ready, less afraid *(of lung cancer)*. I have faith in just about everything I do. I know it will be OK because even if it's not OK, and if it's imperfect, everything is always just going to be right.

Relationships with Family, Friends, and Acquaintances

(When) any of my friends or my family heard that I had lung cancer, I think they were very frightened because of the first time *(multiple myeloma)* and seriousness of that. Everyone was here with me— family came down. My husband is a wonderful man. He's very caring. If anything, I got more attention than I usually do. There were better relationships with my family because they understood that it was my second time around *(prior cancer was multiple myeloma)* and they were very concerned about how serious this particular lung cancer was. They didn't abandon me. They loved me throughout it.

Through the recovery we were alone in Florida. Our son and his wife came from the northeast to visit one time. It would have been better and sweeter if the kids were nearby. My husband was my only caretaker. Although under pressure, *(my husband)* cooked the healthiest meals, and our laundry was always ready-to-wear. No complaints from me—lots of love for him.

Satisfaction with Medical Care During Treatment

The lung surgeon was outstanding. When the left lower lobe was removed, I began to have pretty bad chest pains. The nurse was shocked. He called them back and he gave me a nerve ablation *(portion of the nerve is removed to reduce the pain)*. They took *(the pain)* away—it never came back.

My treatment team included experts in cancer care. That's their focus—nothing else—it's cancer care. The cancer specialist at *(the cancer center)* took my recovery as personally as I did. The first thing that struck me was the way the staff interacted with one another. You can see that they really liked each other. You come in the *(hospital room)* and wonder if the girl standing there was my sister, because she was always there. She was the nurse. Oncology nurses are very special. They take ownership of your life and body. I was in pain in bed. My doctor said: "Go and take a shower. You're going to feel better. That's what I tell my wife." He was this home-like family.

PATRICIA12345: *Lung Cancer, Stage I, 77 years old, female, disease-free 3.5 years; Prior cancer: Breast Cancer*

Life One Year Before Diagnosis

I had breast cancer and had a lumpectomy and radiation in 2013. *(However)*, before I was diagnosed with breast cancer, it was like life was just going on. I was doing all my volunteer work and there was not too much stress in my life at all.

Diagnosis of Lung Cancer

It was during radiation for breast cancer when they found this spot on my left lung. They kept an eye on it for a year. Every three months I would have a CT scan and after a year, they determined that whatever it was, it had to come out. It was determined to be lung cancer. When I found out that they had to remove it and were going to separate my ribs, I did become a little bit antsy about the surgery. My first concern was, "Is it going to hamper my activities because I live alone?" I do my own housework, I move my own furniture, I do everything myself. I did become concerned what the surgery was going to be like. I never felt that it was any more than just going in and having your gallbladder taken out or appendix taken out. That's all it was. I lived my life for years and years where I was pessimistic because I guess we had so many things happening when I was young. I thought, "Why get excited about this, because something else is going to happen?"

The first thing people started asking me was, "Is this because of you smoking?" It didn't offend me. I said, "I quit a long time ago. The doctors said "No. *(It was not because of my smoking)*." If you say the doctors said "No," people believe the doctor before they believe me.

Treatment and Treatment Side Effects

The surgeon removed 80% of my lower left lung lobe. My oncologist determined that I was going to need chemo, and my radiologist said, "No chemo during radiation." I was 72 years old; I felt really healthy. I can't see putting poison in my body that's going to make me sick for a year. So, I decided I just didn't want any further treatment." My oncologist was sitting there with his arms folded and he was really listening to me and, after I finished he said, "I think you've made a very wise decision." I just felt that I had these surgeries, they just interrupted my busy schedule, and I just got on with my life. I had no further treatment after that. I think that at the end of two weeks, I was out and about as if nothing had ever happened.

Quality of Life During Treatment

Relationships with Family, Friends, and Acquaintances

I didn't get any support from my family when I had breast cancer (*13 months prior to having lung cancer*). (*When I was diagnosed with lung cancer,*) my oldest daughter came and spent the night with me one night. She brought my grandson with her. I really enjoyed their company. My grandson was probably about four and so he would like to get something for me and said, "Grandma, can I get you this or can I get you that?" So, I had good support from them. I really felt fortunate for all the support from everybody.

I had a lot of support from all of my friends as well. They were all wanting to bring me food. They would call me. They would send me emails. I'm still in the book club of a group of friends in Dearborn (*where I had lived*). My friend Rose had it all scheduled so that somebody was here with me every day the first week I was home from the hospital. One of them stayed overnight the first night and then the next night my daughter Trisha came over and stayed. But, then I told them all I was fine being here by myself because I knew I could just make a phone call to a neighbor if I needed something. Just having my friends be here, not so much doing stuff, but just having them, knowing that they all wanted to come and help, it was a wonderful feeling. I just felt so grateful.

Coping with Having Cancer

Having an active lifestyle is what kept me going. I didn't stay home and feel sorry for myself because I figured that nobody else is going to feel sorry for me. So I might as well get out amongst the living, so I kept active.

Satisfaction with Medical Care During Treatment

I was very pleased with the surgeon I had. I thought I got wonderful care in the hospital and I've used that hospital for all of my medical care.

WARREN: *Lung Cancer, Stage II, 78 years old, male, disease-free five years*

Life One Year Before Diagnosis

Since retirement, I've been doing the same thing as I've been doing for 20 years. Life was very peaceful. I am diabetic, but it's very mild. A year or two before *(my diagnosis of lung cancer)* I had some trouble breathing in completely.

Diagnosis of Lung Cancer

In August 2012 I scheduled an appointment with my doctor to see if maybe there's something that I need to look at—what this having trouble breathing was about, because I really should be able to breathe in. In September I had an X-ray. My doctor said, "It appears that there's some shadow on your lungs and I'd like you to come in and we'll examine it more closely." When I came in, he said, "This looks like it's a tumor." I thought it could be nothing or it could be something and if it's something, it could be treatable or it could be untreatable. I was very equanimous about it. Then I went in and the doctor said, "It's a slow-growing tumor. It's Stage II." I don't know why I have this tumor. I don't smoke, I'm healthy, I work out three times a week, I go hiking 6 to 10 miles up and down mountains.

Treatment and Treatment Side Effects

(After the surgery,) my doctor said, "We wound up removing the upper third of your right lung. It will grow back or parts of the alveoli *(tiny air sacs in lung where the mixture of oxygen and carbon diox-*

ide take place) will grow back. It will gradually seal the empty space there." I was in the hospital for five to seven days. After surgery, there was shortness of breath, but that was because my lungs were rebuilding after surgery. There was no pain. MRIs were done every three or every six months, as the doctor was looking for anything that might indicate that the lung cancer had spread. Follow-up exams became yearly trips. Then after five years it stopped.

Quality of Life During Treatment

Relationships with Family, Friends, and Acquaintances

My wife is my best friend. I'm her best friend. She's all the emotional content that I need in life. *(When we took a trip to Brazil, we got robbed of our passports and money).* We just looked at each other and said, "OK, what's the next step?" That's how we did it. That's been true all through the 40 years of marriage. My relationship with my oldest son, his wife, and their daughter is very good. They're a great family and they like to spend time up here. My middle son is eccentric. We communicate with him mostly by email. Occasionally we'll go out to see him, but he never comes down to see us because he doesn't like the city. Our relationship with our youngest son is peculiar because he's just odd. He has always been odd and marched to his own drumbeat. I don't really have friends. I don't get anything from social interactions. I'm perfectly happy being alone.

(Friends never said that it was my fault in getting lung cancer.) They said that it was just bad luck—you don't smoke, you exercise, you're not overweight. None of the markers or the usual causes were operational.

Coping with Having Cancer

I have a really good defense mechanism which kicks in whenever there is a problem. Sixty years of meditation has done its job. Every single problem that my wife and I have had, we just deal with it in a matter-of-fact way. You just take it a step at a time. Before I got lung cancer, my wife had breast cancer—we handled it. We weren't blown out of the park or particularly frightened by the possibility that she might die. Now she's cancer-free.

Satisfaction with Medical Care During Treatment

My medical care was A1. I was optimistic that the doctor would be capable and that things would go well, and indeed they did. That optimism comes from feeling I've been very lucky in life.

SHERRY H.: *Lung Cancer, Late Stage III or IV, 82 years old, female, disease-free 2.5 years*

Life One Year Before Diagnosis

I felt pretty good *(the year before I was diagnosed with lung cancer)*. I was outside every day. I belonged to three orchid clubs. I looked forward to going to these orchid clubs.

Diagnosis of Lung Cancer

I had problems with breathing. I just thought it was my asthma that I had in my teens coming back. When I thought I had asthma and trouble breathing, I had fatigue. You're worn out trying to breathe. I also had pneumonia in 2009 and I was constantly getting bronchitis. I went to a pulmonary doctor. Finally, the pulmonary doctor sent me to the hospital to take a couple of tests and she said, "I hate to tell you, you have lung cancer." I always fear bad news. *(Having had rheumatic fever for five years when I was a child (5–10 years old), and lupus as an adult for six years, ending in 2002, and been cured of both),* I really thought, right from the beginning, that I beat everything else, I will beat this. *(But)* I had the feeling that my family thought I was going to die.

Treatment and Treatment Side Effects

Chemo never bothered me at all. I hated the radiation. It is, by far, the worst thing I went through. It's hateful. Laying on the table, which is hard as rock, and being naked waist up in an air conditioned, freezing cold room, is just miserable. It apparently burned my chest. To this day it itches. I put cream on it—it doesn't work. Radiation caused my heartburn. The doctor gave me prescription pills that were useless. My neurologist gave me a liquid medication that worked. The heartburn ended. Fatigue was my middle name. I don't know how much chemo caused it, but I was fatigued during both radiation and chemo. Terrible. Due to having had lupus, I developed Sjogren's Syndrome, *(autoimmune disorder causing decreased tears and saliva, which can be complicated by infections of the mouth, resulting in tooth decay)*. The doctors had to remove all of my teeth. I had dentures for two weeks when I was diagnosed with lung cancer. I lost 47 or 48 pounds due to having radiation, and haven't put weight back on. *(Consequently)*, the dentures did not stay because when you lose that much weight the dentures will not fit. Eating is a problem. I can't eat anything that requires heavy-duty chewing. My daughter from California is now living in my rental house and I'm not collecting the rent that I used to. *(So)*, I can't afford to go back to take care of the teeth right now. *(It makes me feel)* terrible.

Quality of Life During Treatment

Functioning

(Chemo and radiation affected my doing my everyday activities) a lot. I didn't go anywhere. I was mostly watching TV. My daughter that lives here in Florida at that time would come over with her boyfriend. I was glad that she left because I couldn't sit there and do polite conversation. I wanted to go to bed.

Relationships with Family, Friends, and Acquaintances

Everybody in the family and anybody I talked to continually said that *(I had lung cancer because I smoked for 45 years)*. The pulmonologist told me it was my fault. It did not upset me. I had to agree with them—I was a bad smoker. *(However,)* that slowed down when more written material was available and it was on TV about people who get lung cancer had never smoked a day in their life.

I would be going to radiation at one location and to chemo at a different location. "How was I going to go to these two different locations?" I was told that I was going to have to find somebody that is going to drive me to my doctor appointments at these two locations. One daughter lived in California and the other one had been divorced and was living with a boyfriend in Florida at that time, and also not about to give up her life. I was stuck with finding somebody that was going to drive me. I asked a friend who lived next door if he could drive me. He was willing to do anything. He lives with me now and he is my best friend. I would depend on him if I needed anything—he would jump in and just do it. I have one girlfriend here. I became very close to one of my tenants, but she works all the time. She and her husband come over once a week. I don't have a whole bunch of friends.

Financial Problems

I had Medicare and the AARP supplement. It got more expensive and I couldn't afford it. I had to give it up even before the cancer. I switched to Medicare Advantage and that paid for my original doctors. They have seen me through everything and they belong to that particular plan. However, I paid a lot of bills for the poisons *(chemo medications)* which were in excess of what Medicare Advantage would pay for. There were also copayments for seeing heart and neurology specialists. I don't have a large Social Security and I couldn't increase the rent on the best tenants I ever had.

Satisfaction with Medical Care During Treatment

I didn't like the radiation oncologist. I didn't like what he had to do to me. He didn't provide information that I felt would be useful. (*I liked the*) medical oncologist. He answered questions. If I asked for written materials, I got them. When you've seen as many doctors as I have in my lifetime, and a lot of them are useless, then you start looking for information, sometimes in desperation. Sometimes I have to ask other people in order to get the information that I want.

GIL: *Lung Cancer, Early Stage, 85 years old, male, disease-free five years*

Life One Year Before Diagnosis

Emotionally, I was not feeling bad at all. I'm a pretty light-hearted guy. Not too many things bother me. I have a very close relationship with my family. All my family was here in the Boca Raton area (*where I live*), and I was able to see them quite a bit. My wife was a brilliant woman who had migraine headaches all the time and used pain killers exclusively. They caused a problem with her blood vessels and she passed away. I lost a great companion when I lost my wife. When I moved to Boca Raton I met a young woman and I started a nice relationship with her. The sad part is that she has dementia now.

Physically, I was in pretty good shape. I went to a vascular surgeon and I found out that I had clogging of the arteries of my leg. The doctors put some bypass stents in to correct that, which has helped a great deal. When I came to Boca Raton, the first thing I had done was a triple bypass surgery on my heart. So far, no problems with that. I also had difficulties in walking and I have spinal stenosis, but that had no effect on my life. I was just a little stiff when walking.

Diagnosis of Lung Cancer

I started coughing and spitting up some blood. The pulmonologist examined me and I had a couple of X-rays done and he saw something. He referred me to a pulmonary surgeon who removed a little section of the tumor and it was diagnosed as lung cancer. When they told me that I had cancer, I was really not that upset.

Treatment and Treatment Side Effects

The tumor was encapsulated *(had not spread to other parts of the body)*, so I did not need radiation or chemotherapy. That was a great relief. *(Having been diagnosed and treated for lung cancer)* didn't affect me that much. My feelings are if you catch cancer early enough, you can cure it. Thank God it worked out fine.

Quality of Life During Treatment

Relationship with Family, Friends, and Acquaintances

I was able to deal with *(having lung cancer)* myself. I would speak to my kids and they were very comforting. I spent a week at my lady friend's house after I was discharged from the hospital, and then I came home and I was fine. I live by myself, and I take care of my home very nicely, with no problem.

Satisfaction with Medical Care During Treatment

I was very, very satisfied. I had a thoracic surgeon who was super. He had a lousy personality, but he was a great, great doctor. He just wasn't warm. I know he cared about all his patients because he had such a super reputation. But I wanted someone at that time, right after surgery to be cuddly and warm, but he wasn't warm. *(The surgeon said)* "You need to do this, you have to do that, and if you don't you are going to have adverse reactions." I said, "All right," and, that was it. But, he was a wonderful, wonderful surgeon.

AFTER TREATMENT AND THROUGH SURVIVORSHIP

KATHY V.: *Lung Cancer, Stage IB, 68 years old, female, disease-free one year*

Treatment Late Side Effects

(Because my breathing was more labored) I use an inhaler now. But I'm going to get past that. I've now joined a gym, because I'm determined to get my stamina and endurance back.

Quality of Life after Treatment and Through Survivorship

Emotional State

For ten months out of the year, I don't think about it *(having the CT scan)*. One month prior to the month when I have to get the CAT scan, I dwell on it and I get scared. *(In my latest)* scan, there is a slight nodule on my right lung, the other lung. It was expressed to me that my doctor, radiologist, pulmonologist, and oncologist weren't concerned about it, so I should not be concerned about it. Except you've got to get into my brain and make sure my brain also agrees with that. Now I just have that little nudge at the back of my mind. This is the thing that I've always had. You don't want to overtest because you'll see things that are not relevant, and will have no bearing on your health. But when I see the whole body scans *(my doctor)* might find something bad and you'll get all upset. That's really the only thing that's pressing on my mind. *(However)*, if I had to weigh in the worst things, it would be losing *(my husband)*.

Pets: My dog is absolutely a great reliever of stress. She hasn't been doing well and it has made me think what will I do without her.

Relationship with Family, Friends, and Acquaintances

My daughters and I have a great relationship now. After *(my husband)* died, the girls were very protective of me and taking care of me. Then, when I was diagnosed with lung cancer, it has just continued. My oldest *(daughter)* will call me once a week at least, which she never did before. *(My other daughter)* is the one that drove me crazy as a baby, as a young one. They have become more loving, more concerned. As a person who knows I'm mortal, I'm concerned about where are my girls and who's going to take care of me. I think *(my daughter)* would move back home if I were sick. I know both of my sisters would. I also have friends who would.

(Understanding the effect of having cancer has had on my relationships) is murky. It's intertwined with the fact that I've been widowed and my friends are extremely cognizant of that. It's more related to my living alone now than it is to cancer. Although I know that my friends are there for me, it's helped that I have neighbors around me and all I have to do is pick up the phone. I got this chair the other day and had to put it together and I couldn't get it together. So I called my neighbor and it's together now. I do have good people in my life. At church, you know everybody is concerned, but *(having had cancer)* is now on the back burner—it's not on people's minds. That's OK; I'm fine with that. I do have a good support group there and I have neighbors here.

Non-Cancer Stresses

I don't have a caregiver here. I know my girls would do what they could but that is a concern for me when I think long-term and into the future. Just the maintenance of the house and doing things that I've never done before has been stressful. I'm getting better at it. But, now finding somebody who could help me with the house and not having somebody else to help *(has been a stressor)*. All that is tied to losing my husband. I am redoing parts of my house, as my daughter has encouraged me: "Make it yours, Mom." I've taken things down that were up and I'm putting things up that mean more to me or are about me. Being comfortable to begin with helps with loneliness and watching TV in the evening. *(My volunteer and educational activities)* made me just get out there by myself. But it will work out. To me I think you have to talk to yourself and say, "You know what? That's nothing you can control," so try not to stress about it because I can't control it.

Regaining and/or Changing One's Life

I am still struggling with "Who am I now?" I don't really know because my life has changed so drastically, and that's hard. *(After surgery)* I went to my regular doctor and said to her, "Now I have to live my life in six-month segments *(time between doctor appointments)*." She said, "Oh no. You live your life. You don't look at it as six-month segments. You just live your life." There are many days when I don't even think about cancer. So, to me, I feel like I'm coping with it and I'm not dwelling and getting stuck in the mud *(because)* of it. I want to be the way *(my husband)* was, as much as I can—to just deal with it and do what you have to do. Humor was how both my husband and I handled the stress of illness. *(It helped to)* make light of the situation. Sometimes you have to just find what the gallows humor is *(in having had cancer)*.

I'm only now starting to actually get things accomplished. I got the basic things accomplished as far as paying the bills and stuff for the house. I'm starting to rearrange things now, but that again is more in line with not having my husband here. *(My daughter)* said to me, "You need to make this room like the room that I had set up for *(Dad)* your room." So, I'm working on changing things in there. But I could not have done that a year ago, whether it was because of the cancer diagnosis or because I didn't have the energy.

I've reached out to friends more. I'm trying to be more involved in the organizations that I've always been in, *(beginning before I had lung cancer). (In)* my church I was very involved when I was on the board for the preschool that we have. I belong to a women's organization that promotes education for women who want to come back to education. This includes offering some grants to them so they can finish their degrees. Once a week, I do volunteer work at the food pantry.

I am very fortunate to live in an area that offers many programs for people dealing with cancer. Not only support groups, but educational seminars. I went to a couple of seminars, particularly lung cancer, which gave me a lot of information. I need to be intelligent about what's going on with my health. It doesn't mean I'm going to obsess about it, but I do feel I want to know what's going on and what my risk factors are. So, to me, educating myself is important.

Satisfaction with Medical Care after Treatment and Through Survivorship

The pulmonologist's nurse practitioner read the report from the radiologist: "There was a 2 mm ground glass nodule on the right lung, stable." I've never heard that before. I've been trying to call my doctor now to find out. I need my oncologist to tell me when this was first noticed. If it's stable that means that he had seen it before. I've called the nurse twice. She called back once, but of course I was not home. I have to make sure my oncologist realizes that I want all the information. That's what I have to make sure I communicate to him, "Don't try to hide it from me because from now on, I'm going to ask for those reports to be sent to me." Other than that, I feel very good about the medical care I got.

Overall Impact of Having Had Cancer

Negative and Positive Effects

The negative is that I do feel robbed of the freedom of knowing that I'm healthy and that I don't have to worry about things. I feel like, "God, why are you doing this to me?"

I used to feel that I would live a long time and I hope I do. But I feel more vulnerable now with life, which makes me want to not get hung up on the little things, but to appreciate what I have had and who I'm with. That's what's important—really finding out what's important to me. It makes my family more present for me when they come over and I see them. Again, losing my husband also comes into this. I don't ever feel truly happy and that's because even the happy times will have sadness because he's not there to share it. My husband use to say "Faith, family, and friends," and really that's what life is about. As we get older, in particular, when we don't have all the mobility or the health we once had as younger people, it comes down to that.

Advice

Take care of yourself. To love the people you're with. To appreciate the small things. To not obsess about the future. To have faith, that is, if you have it, keep your faith and enjoy your life.

I think it is important for cancer patients/survivors to be open to antidepressants, pain medication, and help with sleeping if they need it. Not all doctors suggest this to their patients, and patients should not be afraid to ask. It is not a matter of being "brave" but of making your life easier to handle.

I've been thinking about how many people tell me that I am strong. I feel it is important for everyone who is coping with cancer to know that: (a) it is not possible to be strong all the time—period—and (b) it is okay to not be strong. To not be strong is not failing, it is human and it is OK.

ISABELLA: *Lung Cancer, Stage IV, 70 years old, female, in remission 1.5 years*

Quality of Life after Treatment and Through Survivorship

Non-Cancer Stresses

I still have arthritis in various joints which is not a huge problem, but because of Tarceva, I can't take any of the arthritis medicines. I have very bad arthritis in my lower back and had to have an epidural early on while I was in treatment, which fortunately has worked for a long time. It's more like regular old age stuff than powerful illness. I also have a son with a terrible brain injury and a heroin addiction which he's not addicted to right now, or is clean at the moment, and another son who's very difficult. That's a euphemism for near-impossible.

I am saved by having worked for Kaiser and having Kaiser insurance. I never had to worry about that. The financial burden is due to having less income, because I can't work. Now, I don't want to work and maybe I could, but I don't want to try. *(More)* money would let me be able to get more household help, so I don't have to yell to get to do things; and more transportation help, so I don't have to do all the driving. On the other hand, compared to everybody else, did we go without or lose our house? No.

Coping with Having Had Cancer

The social worker at the hospital said, "This Cancer Support Community is supposed to be helpful and you should go there." Very reluctantly I did go there and now of course I adore them. I got put in with a group four years ago. We're still like brothers and sisters. We would do anything for each other. If one of them calls that they have a problem, we are there. If somebody is upset about something, we meet for lunch. Was an extraordinary group of people. I do believe we saved each other.

The Cancer Support Community (CSC) #1, provides a strong sense of "you're not alone"; #2, there are people in worse shape than you are; #3, they address the fact that life doesn't stop just because you got cancer. Everybody had other grief going on in their life. We are very protective of one another. I feel if I need support emotionally now, I would turn to my family or CSC. I feel now that I'm not cured *(but in remission)*, and not very ill.

Now I have another job. I volunteer at the kindergarten, I volunteer at the house of justice, helping people fill out papers for their kids in case they got deported—"What will happen to the children?" I volunteer with the people at the Cancer Support Community and I help by giving out information for the Lung Cancer Foundation. In all of them I'm appreciated, more than I ever was in my own job.

Coping Needs That Went Unmet

I have one spectacular cousin who came out immediately after I was diagnosed and went with me to the accountant and the lawyer to help me *(put my affairs in order)*. More of that kind of family help would have been lovely, but everybody is dead.

Satisfaction with Medical Care after Treatment and Through Survivorship

I have a different oncologist now who is more knowledgeable about lung cancer. I had a second opinion from a big specialist which was very helpful. I was very happy with him. He will be available to me if I need him in the future.

Overall Impact of Having Had Cancer

Negative and Positive Effects

If I have one huge complaint it's that I want more energy. It's really very difficult for me to go out at night even for something easy. I quit the choir at the temple because I was just too tired. That's part of the thing everybody says that that's a "new normal." "This is your 'new normal'—shut up and deal with it" and I am able to do that.

Some of the negatives are the reactions from people who don't "get it"; the reactions from people who think you are dead and you're walking around. "So why aren't you doing this or why are you still tired? If your cancer's in remission why can't you come to choir or do XYZ?" I don't think people understand that we're not the same as we were before diagnosis and before treatment. Fortunately, it doesn't piss me off or get me really agitated or anything. It's like I'm too busy and too tired to explain.

The negatives are that during the course of having had cancer you meet so many lovely people online, at the Bonnie J. Addario Lung Cancer Foundation, Cancer Support Community, Inspire which is an online community, and Facebook groups. And then they start to die. In the lung cancer community it's a bunch of 30-year-olds, a bunch of people with little children. The positive is knowing them and the negative is losing them.

The benefits are a greater appreciation for small things, the ability to notice small things, the ability to stay in the present. If my grand-daughter makes a sleep face or does a sleep gesture *(to indicate when she's sleepy)*, I always enjoy that. I can live in that moment a little longer, in that sleepy moment. I never was a person without gratitude. I always appreciated having food on the table and the good things in life. I think I savor it more. I have learned to let go of things that aren't important, not taking stupid things too seriously, not caring what other people think about your house or what you're wearing or what your kids are wearing.

Greatest Concerns

My greatest concerns are the mess that will occur with my grand-daughter if I die. Her parents are inadequate. I also hate feeling like the sword of Damocles hangs over my head. When will it recur? Will I get brain mets *(additional tumors, short for "metastases")*? Become disabled?

Advice

Do things for other people: volunteer, help a kid learn to read, do something. You can lie around, just don't lie around 24/7. Find somewhere to volunteer that is something you really enjoy and that's physically not taxing. Every elementary school probably in the country could use people to help kids who are struggling with reading and this, that, and the other. So many people could do that. There're just lots of things you can do.

SUSAN OS: *Lung Cancer, Stage IIIA, 71 years old, female, disease-free one year*

Long-Term Treatment Side Effects

(One of the side effects is problems with my memory.) If I go to a movie or play, I have difficulty following what's going on. I may have forgotten what I was reading after reading, but, as I'm reading, I comprehend everything. I don't get lost going any place, stuff like that. I'm going for memory help at *(the cancer center)*, but I don't think it's doing very much. I accept *(having memory problems)* because there isn't much *(the cancer center)* can do about it.

Another side effect is neuropathy in the bottom of my feet. It is not painful at all, but I've noticed that my balance is not as good as it has been. I don't know if that will ever go away. When I say my balance is bad, I don't mean walking in the street. I mean doing advanced yoga poses. When I go to a yoga class at the gym every Sunday, I see that I'm stronger every Sunday. I can't do the most difficult classes in the gym that I've attempted. I think there was one class that was very tough, and I haven't done that one. But I've done all the others. I also get out of breath much more easily than I had been, which is to be expected. They took out a big piece of my lung.

Quality of Life after Treatment and Through Survivorship

Coping with Having Had Cancer

What helps me cope is having a loving husband and being able to do the things I enjoy doing. If I can go to the gym, which, believe it or not, I enjoy doing; *(I also enjoy)* being with people, being with my friends, going out to dinner. I really can't say that any of it *(having had cancer)* was so difficult. I think the reason for that is when I was in the hospital, I saw other people who had great difficulty in moving around. I could do everything that I did before, other than, of course, getting out of breath more easily. I can outperform most people who are much younger *(than I am)*, even now.

Prior Issues That Affected Coping

I think I was used to having bad things happen. I was 15 years old when my mother died and my father wasn't around a lot. He went to work in the morning and didn't come home until late at night. I was virtually on my own at that time. Since I had bad things happen in the past and I got through it, I said, "All right. This is another bad thing. I'll get through this one too."

Overall Impact of Having Had Cancer

Negative and Positive Effects

(I have) the memory problem, the shortness of breath upon intense exercise. I wouldn't say there's anything positive that comes out of this.

Greatest Concerns

My greatest concern is if it's going to come back. *(The fear)* is always there. It obviously gets worse a couple of days before the scan. It's not an intrusion *(on my life on a daily basis)*. It's just like an unpleasant feeling. It's not preventing me from doing anything that I want.

Advice

Go to a *(major cancer center)*. Do everything your physicians order. Call them if anything seems problematic. Be optimistic. Keep exercising.

CHERYL L.: *Lung Cancer, Stage I, 72 years old, female, disease-free three years; Prior cancer: multiple myeloma*

Quality of Life after Treatment and Through Survivorship

Emotional State

The lung cancer surgery was a simple procedure and the doctor was wonderful. I remembered, of course, the terror of the multiple myeloma diagnosis *(prior cancer)*. But it was easier because of that to accept this *(lung cancer)*. When I finished with the whole treatment and came home, my husband had a little puppy in the house for me. That was a blessing. My first oncologist asked me: "Have you ever thought about what you would do if you relapsed?" And my answer was: "No, not really." I guess, instinctively, I protected myself by not having to go to a worry mode every three months *(when I had a scan of my lungs)*.

Relationships with Family, Friends, and Acquaintances

My husband and I could never stop being affectionate with one another. However, my back has definitely curtailed some action. *(My sexual life)* has slowly gone and my husband is very considerate of it. I don't think that either one of us feel a big loss in that area. My family, my son Paul and his four kids and wife, they just didn't realize *(how cancer affected me)*. When they came down to visit with me, they saw me in living color. I have a few relatives that are exceptional. My daughter-in-law—we call her our daughter—she's good as gold. She just watches out; she calls me and pays attention. She doesn't miss a trick.

What's on my mind right now is that people didn't understand *(how I was doing)* until they saw the way I was walking and the limitations that I had, how many times I fell and broke my fingers, and that I broke my foot. They just didn't understand unless they went through their own serious illness. But I have very close friends. For many years they came to visit with me. They really pay attention to what I'm saying.

Other Medical and Nonmedical Stresses

My son Jeffrey passed away. That was the worst thing; nothing compared to that. While that was happening, my father couldn't hear a thing. I was very close to Dad, but I couldn't cope with him—he was too sick and died within a year. *(My husband)* carried the whole ball. One of my cousins, a delicious cousin, died last year. He was very, very good to my children. A month ago, I lost another cousin. He kept the family together—he was a wonderful person. I'm very lonely for people who are no longer here. I've never lost that feeling of loneliness. But there is much more to be grateful for. My husband knows what I needed.

After the lung cancer and back surgery *(not lung cancer-related)*, it set me back a lot; not in my mind, but in my body. The chronic back pain inhibits much of what I do, such as dancing, walking, standing too long. I'm fine emotionally, except for the fact that my back is so bad and I am very limited in how long I can stand or walk. That gets me down. I know I have been talking to my friends and people who have had the same experience, and it helps. I can't go on vacation, not until I find some solution *(to the back pain)*. The steroid shots and epidural shots didn't do a thing for me. I did physical therapy I think for three months and it was very good, but the pain just kept getting worse. Even though I had back surgery, frankly, it didn't do one thing to help me. I met a doctor here who specializes in pain management. He offered me stem cell therapy. It is my last chance really. I don't know what else to do. I've done everything I can for this back.

In the past five years, in addition to my chronic back pain, I also had broken ribs, pneumonia, bronchitis, the flu, a broken foot, and digestive problems. Two weeks ago, I was so sick—I couldn't stop coughing. I didn't want to be alive. The *(medical problems)* were so endless. But I'm not going to stop.

Satisfaction with Medical Care after Treatment and Through Survivorship

I was blessed with a special treatment team. Ultimately, I was filled with hope. My oncologist is right on the money with everything.

She does not forget to look at various things in my life that might contribute to a relapse or other problems. She is so kind. She would call me with the results of the test. She would call me at home, rather than having the assistant call me. I find that very touching.

Overall Impact of Having Had Cancer

Negative and Positive Effects

There were no negative effects. The positive about it is that I'm OK. The second *(positive)* is that I can talk to people about the fact that I'm in remission and that *(the cancer)* was caught early. I am left with an immense amount of gratitude by supporting *(the cancer center's)* world-class cancer research. One of the reasons that I volunteer and get so involved is because, as a patient, I know that I can't underestimate the value of what donors can do because they keep the progress going. *(Through volunteering to serve in cancer organizations,)* maybe I'm giving some hope to people. That has been what my life has turned into: my public speaking and speaking to support groups. I speak to people one-to-one on the phone who have been referred to me from the Leukemia and Lymphoma Society or from the Jewish Family Services where I volunteer. That's the only thing I know I can do now. I've been doing it for a long time, for 11 to 12 years. That's my job in life. The patients and survivors don't go it alone because you are not alone; that's what saved me initially. When I went to the Wellness Community support group, it was everything. I had friends who had the same disease; they gave us information about insurance. You can see the reaction of someone who knows exactly what you're feeling—that's priceless. The Wellness Community has asked me to write a column every quarter in their newsletter. The heading is: "<u>My Imperfect Journey: A Quarterly Journal by Cheryl L</u>." I'll be able to say things that I think would be important to somebody. They will help somebody who's suffering due to any cause. I want people to understand that this is the best way I can give to make myself well. I really believe that this is also physically very important to my body. All the volunteering— it keeps me going.

Greatest Concerns

I am more fearful of my back pain being unending than of relapsing with cancer. The most important issue for me now is becoming pain-free. When am I going to be able to live my life?

Advice

You have to be the master of your own treatment team. Be attentive about how your treatment team treats your body and your mind. I know that if I'm not vigilant in the way I ask my treatment team to take care of me, they could miss something and I wouldn't be aware of it, and then I'd be in trouble. You have a choice of any doctor that you wish to go to, but you want the doctor to be qualified. It's your job to be master of your fate. Of all the forces that make for a better world, nothing is so powerful as hope. With hope, one can think, one can dream. If you have hope you have everything.

PATRICIA12345: *Lung Cancer, Stage I, 77 years old, female, disease-free 3.5 years; Prior cancer: Breast Cancer*

Quality of Life after Treatment and Through Survivorship

Emotional State

I never thought of myself as a survivor from cancer. It was just an interruption of my busy schedule. I learned through years of counseling to just stop worrying about what's ahead. Just focus on what's now. I don't worry about what the doctors might find.

Non-Cancer Stresses

The biggest stress in my life has been my three children. By the time my son was 15 years old we found out he was skipping school, he was smoking pot. We took him to a rehab program and then an after-hospitalization program. He dropped out. A year and a half after that *(about 20 years ago)* my husband had a massive heart attack. About two and a half years later he died. After my husband died, I gave each of my children some money so that they could find a place to live. I told them they could no longer live with me. It was just utter chaos with them all together. I haven't seen my son since 2008. He wants nothing to do with me. Every day I lived with the fear that my son might come home with a temper or drugs. *(But)* I miss him. It would be nice to see him, but I can't let my life be defined by my children.

Effect of Prior Cancer on Survivor's Life

When the doctors went to scan my body before radiation *(the treatment that began when I had breast cancer)*, that was when they found the spot on my lung. They watched that for a year. They just didn't know what it was. Every three months I'd go for a CAT scan. At the end of a year, they realized it had doubled in size and they said it would have to come out. That's when they found out it was a malignancy in my lung. That's why I feel if I had not had the breast cancer, the lung cancer could have become severe before I would ever have known.

Coping with Having Had Cancer

I don't very often have a down day and I'll tell you why I say this. It's because years ago when I was in counseling and especially after my husband died, I made it a point to have something on my calendar every day. I had a purpose to do something every day. In 2006, when I was in my 60s, I started taking art classes and now I've become an artist. Beginning in 2005 I joined the Assistance League, a nonprofit thrift store organization. I have never worked so hard in my life. I have done hours and hours and hours of volunteer work for this organization. I'm also active in my church. I help to do everything.

Some Sundays I'm a lector and help with communions. I am on the counting team for counting the collection. I am in a group called Companion Ministry at church, where we go to visit people who are sick. When I go to visit them, I come home and I think, "I am so fortunate to have the life I have compared to these people." I am on the funeral committee at church. People think that it is a hardship for me, but it's my way of giving back because people have done it for my family.

Overall Impact of Having Had Cancer

Advice

You have to make sure you have a good medical doctor. When I first got diagnosed with either breast or lung cancer, one of the ladies in my book club said, "I really think you should go over to *(another medical center)* to get another opinion." I said, "I've been to my primary doctor who knew that I had a lump in my breast. I've got a good surgeon. Why should I go?" I would say get your second opinions if you're leery of what you've been told by the first doctor. If you have confidence in your doctors, I mean trust them, then there's no need to get a second opinion.

WARREN: *Lung Cancer, Stage II, 78 years old, male, disease-free five years*

Quality of Life after Treatment and Through Survivorship

Regaining and/or Changing One's Life

I just gradually eased back into a workout routine, a hiking routine, a biking routine. It was so gradual that nothing stands out as being particularly traumatic. My breathing is back and hiking is back and everything's fine.

Coping with Having Had Cancer

I'm just cognizant of how lucky I have been and how fulfilling my life is. I can't say there was anything that I would think of as traumatic. I don't know where my inner strength came from. I was just accomplished. I was a physicist and used to work in head and neck surgery. I usually wound up doing well and getting spotted for it. Perhaps the knowledge was what made problems less awesome to me.

I am a Buddhist and it's been a significant help to me for 60 years. Buddhism definitely provided serenity and equanimity. I am a believer in both karma *(bringing upon yourself your fate in future existences based on what you've done in your past existences)* and dukkah, which roughly translates to suffering in life that is brought about by clinging to things you might have done in the past, such as clinging to your youth, your good looks, or aversion to anything, such as "I can't stand tall people." If you don't cling to things, you're not frustrated.

Overall Impact of Having Had Cancer

Advice

I don't think I have any advice. Everybody is unique. Those people with a religious background who believe in God, they should try to draw strength from whatever their faith will provide them. Those people who are atheists need to find something else.

SHERRY H.: *Lung Cancer, Late Stage III or IV, 82 years old, female, disease-free 2.5 years*

Quality of Life After Treatment and Through Survivorship

Non-Cancer Problems

Breathing is still a problem in the heat. When I'm at home, I have central air conditioning, so I only have problems breathing when I overexert myself. It is 100 degrees outside now *(in Florida)*, and I have to depend on my friend who lives with me if there is something that's supposed to be done. Asthma has also come back. I'm very limited right now. During the winter, I am out much more. I've also had some bladder problems. I started urinating every two hours. I had a cystoscopy. I do get fatigue a little bit, but it is never like it was. *(Because of the breathing and fatigue problem)* I had to give up growing orchids and going to the orchid clubs. Before I had these problems, I was growing 200 or more orchids. It's breaking my heart, but I feel I'm too weak—it's a big job. *(The financial problems I have now include)* needing to pay my monthly bills and $500 to buy a generator *(because of the heat in Florida)*. I don't know how I'll get it, but I will get it. I stopped going to the orchid clubs, going out to have drinks, and donating things. My mind is clouded with what I need to do. I don't think about anything else.

Coping with Having Had Cancer

Not a whole lot *(of coping with having had cancer has occurred)*. One daughter has been living here for five months and started to get the idea that she's not going to take care of me. That started to sink in. But I felt I would get through this *(having had cancer)*. Cancer is just another destructive disease that I had that interrupted my life.

Overall Impact of Having Had Cancer

Negative Effects

In the orchid community I was starting to get recognized for a lot of my orchid plants. In the beginning, I got blue ribbons. Due to the fatigue, I lost my strength. I'm not growing orchids anymore. You can't grow orchids and go to chemo and radiation. Growing orchids is a full-time job. I had a lot of friends in the orchid industry, and now I don't have them. I don't go to the club meetings and I don't see my friends; I no longer go to the picnics and meetings. It's gone.

Greatest Concerns

I just hope I don't end up in an old-age home. They are horrible down here *(Florida)* and I don't have any money, I don't have any savings. I have this property which has a mortgage. I also came up with a urinary problem and am getting a cystoscopy examination. I have in the back of my brain that cancer travels. Until I get done with the cystoscopy and the urologist says there is no cancer, I'll be worried.

Advice

Fight! Tell yourself that you're going to beat it. There's a million ways you can fight. Most of the ways have to be in your brain.

GIL: *Lung Cancer, Early Stage, 85 years old, male, disease-free five years*

Quality of Life after Treatment and Through Survivorship

Emotional State

Emotionally I have been fine. I didn't feel alone at all.

Relationship with Family, Friends, and Acquaintances

We are very close, all of us. Every night, on his way home from work, my son calls me to check on me, which I appreciate. It is really nice. Almost every Sunday, I have brunch with my son and his family and I see the other kids all the time.

The few friends that I had in Boca Raton were friends that I had in my life from Miami. I still keep in touch with these old friends. At the Country Club *(in Boca Raton)*, where I belong, I really don't have that many close male friends. I see a lot of people at the country club and I know them all by name. But I'm not that social anymore. I go out with one or two other people once in a while. It doesn't bother me at all.

Other Non-Cancer Medical Problems

My difficulties with walking and spinal stenosis have continued. That bothers me. I had physical therapy *(a while ago)*, which helped a great deal. I stopped because *(my walking)* was fine. I'm going to start going back to physical therapy and *(at the country club)* we have water aquatics every morning, which is wonderful. Both help a great deal.

Coping with Having Had Cancer

What helped me cope the most was that I knew I was going to be cured. I had great faith in my doctor. I was very close to my family and my living son who said, "Don't worry, everything is going to work out Dad." And, I was busy. I go to the gym every single morning, I go swimming, I go do water aquatics and then I have another place called "Young at Heart," which is stretching to music, things like that. Then once a week I go to meditation. So, whole mornings are all occupied and afternoons I pick my grandchildren up and drive them home a couple of times a week. So, I will keep busy. *(Having had lung cancer)* didn't really bother me that much.

Overall Impact of Having Had Cancer

Negative and Positive Effects

(Having lung cancer) absolutely did not change my life in any way. The positive effect is that it makes you more cognizant of anything going wrong. I am very friendly with doctors. If I see something going wrong, something that's starting to kick up, I run to a doctor. I'm not afraid.

Greatest Concerns

I want to live a halfway decent life to see my oldest granddaughter get married. I want to see my kids grow up and live a normal healthy life for the next couple of years.

Advice

Don't go in with a defeatist attitude. Go in with a positive attitude and have faith in your doctors—I think that's a plus. Live every day the best you can. Keep occupied. That's the most important thing.

Conclusion: What Older Cancer Survivors Are Telling Us About Having Had Cancer

How Did Older Cancer Survivors Cope with Having Had Cancer

Overview

The age of older cancer survivor participants for the book ranged from 67 years old to 88 years old. In fact, 12 out of 38 participants in this book were 80 years old or older, often referred to as the "older-old", at the time of the interview. The overall purpose of this book is to reduce cancer patients' and survivors' feeling of aloneness, of not being understood, by providing the narratives of the experiences of other older cancer survivors who have gone through exactly what they have gone through in coping with having cancer. By focusing the book on older cancer survivors, men and women who have had colorectal, non-Hodgkin lymphoma (NHL), bladder, or lung cancer, it increases the likelihood that their experiences will be similar to yours with these diagnoses.

It is no surprise that the driving force of older cancer survivors in feeling that they can regain the quality of their lives, is being diagnosed at an *early stage of cancer* that frequently results in a good prognosis. When that is linked with having *excellent medical care*, which almost all of the participants in the book had, it increased survivors' feeling that they have a chance of winning this battle with cancer, of regaining their quality of life, of "landing on top." Without having a very encouraging cancer diagnosis, effective treatments, and excellent medical care in place, getting to the top of that hill will be much more difficult.

It is important to keep in mind that these are not the only issues that play a role in survivors being able to cope with having had cancer. It was clear from all the older cancer survivors who were interviewed, most participants talked about several other major items that were essential in their being able to cope with having this disease and regaining their lives.

(1) Being able to either continue doing at least some activities after treatment that had been central to their enjoyment in life that they had before being diagnosed with having cancer, or develop new areas of interest to them that provided enjoyment in their lives.

(2) Getting a lot of much-needed help from family members, friends, and neighbors in dealing with having had cancer, whether it was just listening and understanding what older cancer survivors had gone through, or helping them with their daily chores, or getting to medical appointments.

(3) Not having other major medical problems or stresses in their lives, such as financial problems, illness, or deaths of family members or friends, either prior to their having cancer, nor during or after their current cancer treatment ended.

(4) Having already developed a strength, a "fighting spirit," an ability to fight and win battles to overcome serious problems that they had before having had this current cancer. These strengths developed from either having been treated for another cancer before being diagnosed with their current cancer, or having overcome other major problems in their lives, such as serious medical problems, the death of a parent, or being sexually abused in childhood. Having had any of these problems in their lives was almost like a training ground for participants' ability to deal with having had this most recent cancer.

(5) Being significantly helped by their religious beliefs in dealing with having cancer. They not only felt that God would help

them, protect them, and care about them, but in addition, they were grateful for members of their church responding to them with their kindness, concern, and help.

(6) Becoming a member of a cancer support group or finding other cancer patients who had their type of cancer, through the internet, both during and/or after their treatment ended. Participants felt that patients in the support groups, who had the same cancer as they did, "got it," that is, understood what they had gone through.

COPING WITH HAVING HAD CANCER: FROM DIAGNOSIS THROUGH SURVIVORSHIP

Across all four types of cancer, there was a wide range of emotions due to having cancer, from diagnosis through treatment and survivorship: fear, depression, hope, relief. Some participants' emotional reaction to being diagnosed with having cancer changed over time, from diagnosis up to the present. Several participants reported being traumatized upon hearing that they had cancer, which is not an uncommon feeling in many cancer patients. "I was overwhelmed and not totally accepting that I had non-Hodgkin lymphoma, because it just seemed so far out. The hospital, as well as my daughter, gave me some material to read. I had read enough to understand what lymphoma was. So, gradually, I accepted the fact that I had it." (**Barbara G.,** NHL, Stage IV, Grade 1–2, 85 years old, in remission two years).

However, other participants spoke about their having a positive attitude about their diagnosis, a "fighting spirit." **Walter A.,** an older-old survivor (NHL, High Grade, 87 years old, disease-free two years) had a similar reaction when diagnosed with cancer as **Carol R.** (Colon Cancer, Stage III, 78 years old, disease-free 3.5 years): "What's happened in the past, I can't change. What's in front of me, I can change.

I always felt that way. If I was not a fighter, I wouldn't be here." As expected, the fighting spirit in the older-old category was mixed with an expression of having had a good life, and that given their age, the end of their life was not so far away. As **Jack Kinkaid**, a bladder cancer survivor (disease stage not known, 85 years old, disease-free four years) expressed it: "I had no problem *(being told that I had bladder cancer)**. It is what it is, and you just get it taken care of. I was 81 years old at that time. Something's going to get me." Even some of the cancer survivor participants who had advanced stage disease, where prognosis is worse, had this same fighting spirit. However, that being said, not all participants came away from hearing this diagnosis with that kind of strength.

What Affected Older Cancer Survivors' Ability to Cope with Having Had Cancer

Coping with Cancer Treatment

The first major step in patients' battle with cancer is their obtaining excellent medical care; it is an essential part of the driving force in their being able to regain the quality of their lives. As you can see from what participants from each type of cancer have talked about, across all ages and both genders, virtually all had total confidence and trust in their medical care, from their oncologists, nurses, and the entire medical team. Words participants used to describe their care were "excellent," "outstanding," and "incredible." Nurses were described as extremely capable and caring, and were considered to be a very necessary and important part of older cancer survivors' medical care. A number of the participants also mentioned that the high quality of medical care that they had received was largely obtained at large medical and cancer centers, and not smaller community hospitals. They found that in the local hospitals where they were initially diag-

---

*Italicized (slanted) typing is used in parentheses when quoting participants to complete their sentences, in order to make the quotes clearer.

nosed, there were fewer oncologists with sufficient expertise in their type of cancer. However, one participant felt that his medical care at his local hospital was excellent and definitely more convenient to get to than traveling long distances to get to a major medical center. The difference between these two views of where older cancer survivors should go to get excellent care is most likely related to the difficulty of diagnosing and treating a lesser-known cancer.

As mentioned in the beginning of this Conclusion, cancer patients' degree of suffering is likely to be reduced if they were diagnosed with cancer at an earlier phase of the disease. **Gil**, a lung cancer survivor participant (Early Stage, 85 years old, disease-free five years) is a perfect example of the benefit of catching a cancer early, before it has spread: "The tumor was encapsulated, and had not spread to other parts of the body, so I did not need radiation or chemotherapy. That was a great relief. Consequently, having been diagnosed and treated for lung cancer didn't affect me that much." On the other hand, **Steve**, an NHL survivor participant (Stage I, 70 years old, in remission one year) had a much more difficult treatment and serious side effects, resulting in a significant impact on his quality of life: "The treatment made me unbelievably sick. I just didn't leave the apartment very much. I had relapsed on four different treatments. When I was done with the bone marrow transplant, one of the treatments, I was very tired, could hardly move and I had terrible pain from peripheral neuropathy. It lasted at least one month. Doing my little aerobic exercises in the pool has been one of the things that kept me going. I had terrible skin problems throughout all the different treatments. Lyrica, a medication used to treat neuropathic pain, destroyed my skin. During those days I was open to trying anything for my pain, and nothing changed it."

While the quality of older cancer survivors' medical care was largely considered excellent, several deficiencies in their care were raised by several participants: (1) their oncologist didn't have sufficient time to spend on patients, (2) insufficient information was provided about their disease and treatment, (3) their oncologist didn't talk about patients' emotional issues, and (4) their medical center didn't provide support groups for their particular type of cancer.

Relationships with Family, Friends, and Acquaintances

A major factor affecting older cancer survivors' ability to cope with having had cancer is the *strength of their relationships* with family members and friends, as well as how *communication* between the survivor and others affected the strength of these relationships. The importance of support from family and friends in coping with having had cancer is pretty much summed up by **Carol R.** (Colorectal Cancer, Stage III, 78 years old, disease-free 3.5 years): "I had the ideal situation I'd say of support, right there with me. I just strongly feel that that was why I recovered so quickly. My heart goes out to people that don't have that. *I don't know how people do this alone.*"

With the increasing number or severity of non-cancer medical problems and frailty as older survivors aged, some participants talked about their not having enough help from family members, friends, and neighbors. This was particularly true for those who were 80 years old or older, due to a shrinking number of those who had provided support in the past, because of: (a) the deaths and illnesses of their spouse, and (b) friends and neighbors, as well as children and other family members, living too far away to help to the extent needed. Consequently, that feeling of aloneness grew, and with it, fear and depression. **Doris R.** (NHL, disease stage not known, 88 years old, disease-free four years) said: "I'm lucky if somebody calls me once a month. I keep telling my kids, "Why don't you call me?" I do call my brother and we get along really well. I have one good friend—my best friend. There were seven or eight of my friends who sat together in church. Now, they are all gone. They either moved out of the area or just don't come anymore. I sit next to myself. I still don't have the energy to fix a meal. You eat alone. It's hard to eat alone all the time."

Communication

What needs to be in place for a strong relationship between a patient and others, across *all* medical problems, particularly serious ones, is that others understand what the patient is going through, and know what to say and how to say it—that they "get it." Some older cancer survivor participants felt hurt and angry when family members and friends did not understand at all what they've been through—how cancer affected their lives. Some participants were able to continue their relationships with others, who they felt did understand. Other participants felt that too many people really didn't understand what they were going through at all, and therefore didn't want to discuss having had cancer with anyone; it was just too painful. The consequences of that may be that it will either be the end of developing a new relationship, and damage or end a current relationship, even if that relationship had been strong prior to the cancer survivors' cancer diagnosis.

Persons of Color (Minorities): Communication with their Doctors

Dr. Christopher Lathan, an African American lung cancer doctor, who is the Medical Director of Dana-Farber Cancer Institute at St. Elizabeth and Faculty Director of Cancer Care Equity at Dana-Farber Cancer Institute, was interviewed concerning the quality of medical care for persons of color. He discussed what he saw as African Americans' dissatisfaction in the communication between the doctor and African American cancer patients. "They feel the doctor didn't really explain what was happening to them in a way they could understand. Further, they felt that they were not being listened to or valued."

Religious and Spiritual Beliefs that Helped Older Cancer Survivors to Cope with Having Had Cancer

A fair number of older cancer survivor participants, across all four types of cancer, reported that religion was a major factor in helping them get through having cancer. As these participants routinely had gone to church, they had developed a group of friends from the church, their "church family," who cared about them, helped them with chores that they were not able to do, and had prayed for them, particularly at the time of treatment and recovery. The way participants described how important their religion was to them, you could almost see their church friends circling around them, protecting them, offering comfort, praying for them. That, along with their strong belief in God, magnified older cancer survivor participants' ability to cope with having had cancer.

Prior Cancers and Other Medical and Nonmedical Stresses

A number of the older cancer survivor participants spoke about other non-cancer medical problems that had occurred either before being diagnosed with having cancer, or during or after treatment, that had continued up until now. While that was expected to be the case, particularly in those survivors 80 years old or older, it was clear from the interviews that even after all their cancer treatment and any long-term side effects, these non-cancer medical problems sometimes took the place of problems that had been caused by cancer. They had now become the major factors affecting older cancer survivor participants' quality of lives. **Cheryl L.**'s back pain began before she was diagnosed with having cancer, and has continued to be a major problem in her life, up to the present. "The back surgery, which was not related to having lung cancer, set me back a lot. It gets me down that the chronic back pain inhibits much of what I do, such as dancing, walking, and standing too long. My back is so bad that I am very limited in how long I can stand or walk." (Lung Cancer, Stage I, 72 years old, disease-free three years; Prior cancer: Multiple Myeloma)

WHAT HELPED AND WHAT KEPT OLDER CANCER SURVIVORS FROM REGAINING THEIR LIVES AFTER TREATMENT

Some of the older cancer survivor participants needed to make significant changes in their lives, due to having had cancer. Their distress over their lost or reduced ability to do those things they had loved to do before they had cancer was offset by some, by either finding satisfaction in making changes to these activities, or finding totally new activities altogether.

Helping other cancer patients was frequently talked about as a major addition to some of the older cancer survivor participants' lives, not only because it helped others, but because it also helped themselves. Survivors were able to talk with patients, like themselves, about their cancer diagnoses. *It made them feel less alone—better understood.* That is one of the fundamental purposes of the cancer organizations and support groups, as well as this book. The sheer widespread use of support programs throughout the nation shows how valued they are in helping patients cope with this disease.

OVERALL IMPACT OF CANCER ON OLDER CANCER SURVIVORS' LIVES

One of the reasons for older cancer survivor participants having this drive to help other cancer patients stemmed from the fact that a number of them had already been in support groups in organizations or medical centers at the time when they were interviewed. Because they felt significantly helped by these support groups and grateful to medical centers that provided excellent medical care, they now wanted to extend themselves to help other cancer patients cope with having had cancer.

Greatest Concerns in Older Cancer Survivors' Lives During Survivorship

It is common that after treatment has ended and cancer survivors have been informed by their doctor that they are cured, they often have a continuing fear of their cancer coming back, especially at the time of their next follow-up exam. Some survivors became very fearful of their cancer coming back a long time before their follow-up exam. This fear is often expressed by many patients and survivors of any age, as "a sword hanging over their head." As mentioned earlier in this Conclusion, other aspects of older cancer survivor participants' lives can play an important role in how afraid they are of their cancer coming back. Those who have more support from their family and friends, a "fighting spirit," or fewer major medical problems or stresses after their cancer treatment has ended, are likely to be less fearful of recurrence than those without these positive aspects in their lives.

Older Cancer Survivors' Concerns Regarding Their Ability to Function

A number of cancer survivor participants who were now disease-free or in remission, focused their attention on being able to take care of themselves or members of their family, if there was an increase in their medical problems and age. "I think of the consequences of aging: whether I'm going to be able to take care of myself, do the things I need to do to stay in my own home, by myself." (**Milly H.**, Bladder Cancer, Stage II, 70 years old, disease-free four years). "The biggest issue for me, especially initially, was how do I continue to take care of my mom and my aunt, when I can't even take care of myself?" (**Ron**, NHL, Stage IIIA, 72 years old, disease-free four years).

Advice

Many of the older cancer survivors' advice to other cancer patients and survivors is built on their own experiences about what helped them, along with advice as to what *not* to do. Most of the advice that participants gave was spoken with a deep feeling of compassion and caring about other cancer patients' and survivors' lives—wanting to help those with cancer to regain their lives.

As detailed in the book, most of the participants reported that their medical care was excellent, from doctors, to nurses, to the entire medical team. When participants were asked about what advice they would give to other patients, often the first thing mentioned was the importance and, in fact, the necessity of getting excellent medical care at large medical centers that have expertise in treating a wide number of cancers. In addition, a number of participants stated that it was very important for cancer patients to get help from: (a) cancer organizations, often due to the need to talk with other cancer patients, particularly those who have their own cancer diagnosis, so that they wouldn't feel so alone, and (b) family members and friends regarding daily activities and chores, as well as providing some medical care at home, such as changing bandages or driving them to and from medical appointments.

This whole issue is underscored by some of the problems that older cancer survivors have because they feel too uncomfortable talking with others about their having cancer. Consequently, they don't ask for help. This was presented in the Communication section in this Conclusion. The advice one participant gave is expressed in just two sentences: "The worst thing you can do when you're diagnosed with cancer is to isolate yourself. At that moment you have got to reach out." (**Lon**, Colon Cancer, Stage III, 70 years old, disease-free two years). By taking the chance of telling others that they had cancer, they would find those who are helpful. This could result in significantly increasing cancer patients getting the help they need, reducing their distress, and therefore increasing their ability to cope with having cancer.

WHAT NEEDS TO BE IN PLACE TO IMPROVE OLDER CANCER SURVIVORS' QUALITY OF LIFE

Suggestions for Providing Support Programs for Older Cancer Survivors and their Caregivers

Support Groups and Patient-to-Patient Programs

By reading the experiences of other older cancer survivors, it is evident that cancer support programs are now routinely used by many cancer centers, and cancer organizations throughout the nation. The older cancer survivor participants clearly state that it not only helped themselves, but, in turn, others as well, as they reached out to help other cancer patients and survivors *to feel less alone, to feel understood,* and to talk with them about ways of coping with having cancer. Cancer support programs initially began as in-person cancer support groups held in medical centers and cancer organizations. They were then expanded to include cancer support groups conducted over the telephone, as well as patient-to-patient programs, where one patient is paired to another patient or survivor with the same type of cancer. With computers now so widely used, the number of cancer patients who have been helped by psychological and social services provided through the internet have grown exponentially. They now include online support groups and messaging between individual cancer patients, which is akin to patient-to-patient support programs. All these approaches share the same goals: providing that feeling of being cared about, less alone, and better understood.

In addition, as many of these programs are available on the computer to patients at home, at no cost, there is no need for patients to travel to a medical center, cancer organization, or neighborhood center. These are very important "pluses" for helping older cancer patients to maintain their comfort and support by being with other patients. However, the major problem older cancer patients face in benefitting from the use of computers is that they are less likely to own computers and to know how to use them than those who are younger. That was clearly a problem for several of the older cancer survivor participants in this age group, particularly those who are 80 years old or older. Therefore, at this time, computers will not be sufficiently helpful in meeting the psychological and social needs of older cancer patients and survivors. With the increasing number of older cancer survivors, it is essential to take these limitations into account when developing new programs to meet their needs. It is essential that the development of these programs begin *now*.

While many participants said that they got everything they needed to help them cope with having cancer when in the hospital, there were several survivors of each of the four types of cancer in this book who spoke about what was needed while being treated in the hospital, as well as after they had finished treatment. NHL and bladder cancer survivors expressed a need for medical centers or community organizations to have more cancer support programs, with those who had the same type of cancer as they had, held either as a group or with just one patient, as in patient-to-patient programs. These cancer support programs at large medical and cancer centers were sometimes not available even for some of the patients with more common cancer diagnoses. This was even more of a problem for smaller hospitals. Given the success of these support groups and patient-to-patient cancer patient services, there needs to be a greater focus on meeting the needs of cancer patients and survivors with the less common types of cancer.

Caregivers

Virtually everything I've said about support programs being more available to older cancer survivors, applies to their caregivers as well, which include the spouse and/or children, grandchildren, and other family members. The problems of aging of older cancer survivors will likely apply to those caregivers who are of a similar age as the patient. An increasing frailty and number and/or severity of older caregivers' medical problems and functioning will likely affect their ability to take care of their loved one. While these types of programs and services are available to caregivers, they are less common than those provided to cancer patients and survivors. Therefore, support programs provided for patients, need to be increased and broadened to meet caregivers' needs as well. They would increase a caregiver's own ability to understand how cancer has affected their loved one's lives, as well as their own, and guide caregivers in how to help their loved ones. In all likelihood that will strengthen a caregiver's relationship with their loved one, increasing both the caregiver's and survivor's ability to cope with this disease.

Suggestions for Improving the Medical Care of Older Cancer Survivors

As you already know from reading the quotes from the interviews of the participants, almost all of them said they received excellent medical care in every way, from both their oncologists and nurses, and often all other staff at the large medical and cancer centers. However, you also have already read that survivor participants made several criticisms about their medical care. The first problem that patients raised was that oncologists did not have sufficient time to spend with them, which resulted in their having insufficient medical information about their cancer and treatment to make decisions about their care. There is no question that oncologists are stretched too thin, resulting in their not being able to spend more time with their patients to provide them with more medical information. There just aren't a sufficient number of oncologists available to treat the increasing number of cancer patients due to the aging of the population. At this point in time, there is really no good remedy for this problem, other than more individuals deciding to become oncologists to meet the increasing demand. A partial solution is that cancer patients should always be advised to get a second opinion, so at the very least, they know what treatment choices are available, with some information provided for each treatment plan.

The second issue raised by one of the participants about her medical care was that her oncologist did not ask her about emotional problems. This resulted in either no psychological treatment being provided or referrals made to mental health professionals. There are multiple reasons that have been suggested as to why this is happening, in addition to doctors being stretched too thin: (1) oncologists don't feel they know enough about psychological issues to identify those patients who need to be seen by mental health professionals, (2) oncologists feel uncomfortable about talking about these problems with patients, and (3) there aren't a sufficient number of mental health professionals at their medical or cancer center to evaluate and treat patients in need.

A possible solution that might be worth considering is increasing the awareness of both doctors and mental health professionals (psychiatrists, psychologists, social workers) as to the problems and stresses their patients have, in addition to cancer. At the time of their first appointment with their doctor, patients would be given a list of questions (the "Distress Thermometer") about how distressed they are, and what kind of problems they are having: physical problems, emotional problems, and other problems in their lives, such as problems with family and friends (Jacobson et al. 2005). It takes only a couple of minutes to answer these questions. With the patients' permission, this information would then be automatically sent to both their doctor and a mental health professional (psychiatrist, psychologist, or social worker), so that both know what problems their patients face. Patients would then be contacted by a mental health professional to further discuss their distress, and when needed, discuss possible psychological treatments to help them cope with having cancer. This approach might help to reduce the likelihood that older cancer patients' psychological needs would go unmet.

OVERALL THOUGHTS AND WISHES

There is a balancing act of the strengths that many of the participants had—a "fighting spirit," strong relationships with family and/or friends, and strong religious beliefs—which is challenged by problems, such as their cancer being caught at a more advanced disease stage, difficult treatment, other medical problems, less available support from family and friends due to illness or death, and increasing financial problems. Some readers of this book will have these strengths and not too many problems, and will have a greater chance of "landing on top." They will be able to regain some, if not most, of the quality of their life that they enjoyed before this battle with cancer began. What helped many older cancer survivor participants to cope the best was being able to let go of what used to be important to them, that they could no longer do, and find some comfort and happiness with their new life. That's not so easy to do, but many participants in this book did just that. It worked for them. I wish the same for you.

Cancer Centers and Organizations That Provide Treatment and Resources for Cancer Patients and Survivors

Organizations Serving Patients with the Four Cancer Diagnoses Selected for this Book: Bladder, Colorectal, Non-Hodgkin Lymphoma, and Lung Cancer

American Lung Association

55 W. Wacker Drive, Suite 1150, Chicago, IL 60601
(800) 586-4872
lung.org

The American Lung Association provides the following services and resources: (1) health education materials for patients and employers, (2) online and in-person courses and programs about lung cancer, (3) Better Breathers Clubs, which include in-person support groups and educational presentations for patients and family members, (4) online communities on Inspire.com, offering peer-to-peer support, (5) Lung HelpLine and Tobacco QuitLine, both online programs, staffed by medical professionals and counselors to answer patients' questions, and (6) Freedom from Smoking, an in-person smoking cessation program.

Bladder Cancer Advocacy Network (BCAN)

4520 East West Highway, Suite 610, Bethesda, MD 20814
(301) 215-9099
bcan.org

The Bladder Cancer Advocacy Network (BCAN) provides the following online services and resources: (1) an online webinar is available with information concerning bladder cancer diagnosis, treatment, and research, (2) online forums for bladder cancer patients to have discussions with each other, and (3) "My Bladder Cancer Stories" posted on the website about the experiences of bladder cancer patients and family members. (4) In addition, BCAN provides a 24-hour support hotline (888) 901-2226, and in-person bladder cancer support groups held monthly at 24 medical centers across 24 states in the United States and Canada.

Colorectal Cancer Alliance (CCA)

1025 Vermont Avenue NW, Suite 1066, Washington, DC 20005
(202) 628-0123
ccalliance.org

The Colorectal Cancer Alliance (CCA) provides the following resources and services for colorectal cancer patients: (1) a phone (877-422-2030) and online helpline (ccalliance.org/patient-family-support/helpline) to answer patients' questions, provide support, and suggest resources to help them cope, (2) online Support Group Chats, which connect patients, family members, and caregivers, providing support from others who have been through a similar situation, (3) online community where patients, survivors, and caregivers worldwide post a question or share their experiences in CCA's chat room, (4) the Buddy Program, in which a patient is connected with a cancer survivor with the same diagnosis, (5) online videos of patients, oncologists, and other members of the oncology team (RNs, social workers) providing medical information, support, and information concerning quality of life issues, (6) online information materials concerning medical insurance, medical care, legal issues, and financial needs, and other informational resources that can be printed out on patients' computers, and

(7) social media, where patients post comments of their experiences to connect with other patients online: Facebook, LinkedIn, Instagram, YouTube.

GO2 Foundation for Lung Cancer (now includes Lung Cancer Alliance)

1700 K Street NW, #660, Washington, DC 20006
(800) 298-2436
go2foundation.org

The Lung Cancer Alliance provides the following services and resources: (1) online HelpLine providing medical information, referral to qualified medical centers, and answers to questions, (2) educational information provided by publications and materials, websites, and webinars conducted online by experts concerning medical and psychological issues, (3) the Phone Buddy program, a one-to-one peer support in which patients are matched to other patients with the same kind and stage of lung cancer, (4) connecting patients with other organizations providing psychological services conducted by professional counselors (e.g. Cancer Support Community, American Psychosocial Oncology Society [APOS], Cancer*Care*).

Leukemia and Lymphoma Society (LLS)

3 International Drive, Suite 200, Rye Brook, NY 10573
(888) 557-7177
lls.org

The Leukemia and Lymphoma Society (LLS) provides the following services: (1) email and online live chat used to provide information concerning disease, treatment, financial, and employment issues, (2) in-person support groups for patients and family members, (3) First Connection, a peer-to-peer support program, which matches a patient or family member with a trained volunteer based on his/her cancer diagnosis, age, and gender to enable sharing of their cancer experiences, (4) online chats for patients and family members as a means for sharing their experiences with others, and (5) online personal stories of cancer patients' experiences.

Lymphoma Research Foundation (LRF)

88 Pine Street, Suite 2400, New York, NY 10005
(212) 349-2910
LRF@lymphoma.org
lymphoma.org

The Lymphoma Research Foundation provides the following resources and services for those with both Hodgkin and non-Hodgkin lymphoma: (1) a Survivorship Clinic, which provides medical care and referral of patients with psychological problems to either a patient-to-patient support program or a mental health care provider, (2) a phone (800-500-9976), and email Helpline (helpline@lymphoma.org) providing information concerning diagnosis and treatment, as well as referrals to financial and legal resources and insurance help, (3) information resources including disease-specific booklets provided online, or by ordered publications, teleconferences (online and over the phone), educational videos (online), and workshops (in-person), (4) the Lymphoma Support Network patient-to-patient support program which connects a patient with a volunteer who has a similar diagnosis (over the phone and by email (supportprogramhelpline@lymphoma.org)), and (5) online forums for patients to share their cancer experiences with others.

ORGANIZATIONS PROVIDING RESOURCES TO PATIENTS WITH ANY TYPE OF CANCER

American Cancer Society (ACS)

250 Williams Street NW, Atlanta, GA 30303
(800) 227-2345
cancer.org

ACS is a national organization with chapters in all 50 states. A great deal of online information about cancer and many issues specific to cancer patients, survivors, and caregiver/family needs is available on their website. Other resources include: (1) the National Cancer Survivorship Resource Center, currently in development, a collaboration between ACS and the George Washington Cancer Institute, serving survivors as they go from treatment to recovery, including information concerning immediate needs for services and resources, quality-of-life issues, and recommendations concerning clinical survivorship care, (2) the Cancer Survivors Network (CSN), an online community that provides discussion boards, chat rooms, and private emails in which cancer patients and survivors and their families can communicate with each other, (3) the Springboard Beyond Cancer, jointly created by the ACS and the National Cancer Institute, is an online program for survivors that provides information concerning self-management of current cancer-related problems and prevention of new ones, (4) online program, MyLifeLine, which allows patients and survivors to develop their own personal webpages concerning themselves and their friends and family, sharing information about cancer resources, and (5) the National Cancer Information Center (NCIC), which has trained cancer information specialists available by phone and online live chat, providing information and connecting them with services and resources in their communities. Local chapters provide weekly support groups for patients and survivors, family and friends, and workshops such as yoga, exercise, and knitting.

Cancer*Care*

275 7th Avenue, New York, NY 10001
(800) 813-4673
cancercare.org

Cancer*Care* provides the following services, many of which are available online or over the phone: (1) individual counseling, either face-to-face, online, or over the phone, (2) a range of support groups, which include an after-treatment survivorship support group and a support group for adults over 65 years old, (3) cancer experiences written by patients and survivors online, for others to read, (4) educational workshops providing information by experts online (cancer.org/connect) or over the phone, (5) publications, (6) Ask Cancer*Care*, an email helpline (info@cancer.org) where patients and caregivers submit questions to experts, and (7) limited financial assistance for cancer-related costs.

Cancer.Net from the American Society of Clinical Oncology (ASCO)

cancer.net

Cancer.Net was developed by an international organization, the American Society of Clinical Oncology (ASCO), which provides the following online information services for cancer survivors: (1) publications available online and videos of experts providing information concerning a full range of medical, psychosocial, and other quality of life issues, (2) listing of organizations providing resources and services for cancer survivors (e.g. Cancer Support Community, LIVESTRONG Centers of Excellence, Cancer*Care*), and (3) videos of survivors talking about their experiences with having cancer.

Cancer Support Community (CSC)

734 15th Street NW, Suite 300, Washington, DC 20005
(202) 659-9709
cancersupportcommunity.org

The Cancer Support Community (CSC) is a large national organization consisting of 170 locations across 24 states, which has now been extended internationally to Japan, Israel, and Canada. Many of CSC's services and resources are provided online or over the phone, with in-person services provided at the local chapters. Online services and resources include the following: (1) information concerning cancer medical, quality of life, financial issues, and finding clinical trials, (2) the Cancer Experience Registry, in which patients and survivors write about their cancer experiences online for others to read, (3) the MyLifeLine program (described above in the American Cancer Society), and (4) the Living Room, providing online contact with other cancer patients and survivors through message boards. In-person services and resources are provided by the local CSC Centers, including: (a) support groups, (b) educational programs, and (c) the Cancer Transitions Program, which provides information concerning physical, psychological, and practical issues that survivors face once treatment is over. (5) the Cancer Support Helpline, providing direct patient contact with counselors over the telephone (888- 793-9355), a list of resources available through other organizations, and "live chat" (online) with patients and survivors.

National Cancer Institute (NCI)

9609 Medical Center Drive, Rockville, MD 20850
(800) 422-6237
NCI.info@nih.gov
cancer.gov

The National Cancer Institute provides online programs: (1) LiveHelp, available for patients and family members to find information in NCI's publications, (2) availability of publications concerning cancer, treatment, and quality of life issues of patients and family members. Publications specific to cancer survivorship include "Facing Forward: Life after Cancer Treatment," "Facing Forward: When Someone You Love Has Completed Cancer Treatment," and (3) links to services and resources at other organizations, including Life after Cancer Program at Memorial Sloan-Kettering Cancer Center, peer-to-peer support programs through the American Cancer Society and the Association of Cancer Online Resources, and practical concerns through the National Coalition for Cancer Survivorship.

SmartPatients

smartpatients.com

SmartPatients is an online organization that provides an online cancer community specific to many cancer diagnoses, including the four cancer diagnoses in this book (bladder, colorectal, non-Hodgkin lymphoma, and lung cancer). Patients, caregivers, and survivors can post their cancer experiences and their knowledge, post questions, or start conversations on any topic.

CANCER CENTERS WITH SURVIVORSHIP PROGRAMS

The selected medical centers listed below are cancer centers that have developed survivorship programs that provide a broad range of services: post-treatment medical care, psychosocial and quality of life services, and resources specific to the needs of cancer survivors.

Dana-Farber Cancer Institute: Adult Survivorship Program in the Perini Family Survivors' Center

450 Brookline Avenue, Boston, MA 02215
(617) 632-3000
dana-farber.org

The services provided by the Adult Survivorship Program include: (1) identifying and treating long-term and late treatment side effects, (2) support groups and individual counseling on the emotional, mental, social, and spiritual aspects of survivorship, (3) nutrition counseling, (4) exercise classes, (5) the One-to-One Program, which pairs a patient with another patient with the same type of cancer, enabling them to provide emotional support due to their shared experiences, (6) Community Resource Specialists, who find survivorship resources near a survivor's home concerning support groups, financial support, and health insurance and employment rights, (7) an online web page for survivors' stories of their cancer experiences, and (8) social media, where patients post comments to connect with other patients online: Facebook, Twitter, Instagram, YouTube.

Emory University Winship Cancer Institute: Wellness for Living Survivorship Program

1365-C Clifton Road NE, Atlanta, GA 30322
(888) 946-7447; (404) 778-1900
winshipcancer.emory.edu

The Wellness for Living Survivorship Program includes the following services and resources: (1) psychiatrists and social workers providing diagnostic and treatment services for patients experiencing psychological problems, (2) referrals to community resources, (3) a Patient and Family Resource Center (404-778-5286) providing information concerning cancer and services available at the Winship Cancer Institute, (4) nutrition services to help patients and survivors manage their diet, (5) exercise facilities provided to cancer survivors through the collaboration of the Winship Cancer Institute and the YMCA, and (6) social media, where patients post comments to connect with other patients online: Facebook, Twitter, Instagram, LinkedIn, YouTube.

Fox Chase Cancer Center: Survivorship Program

333 Cottman Avenue, Philadelphia, PA 19111-2497
(888) 369-2427
foxchase.org

Fox Chase Cancer Center has the following medical services and resources to meet the needs of cancer survivors: (1) Survivorship Clinics for lung, urinary tract (includes bladder), breast, prostate, and thyroid cancer survivors, consisting of survivorship care plans and wellness education. Survivors of other types of cancer receive survivorship care by doctors, nurse practitioners, and physician assistants in the disease-specific clinics, (2) clinics that focus on medical effects of cancer and its treatment, (3) services for survivors with ostomies, (4) support groups (215-728-2668), (5) psychological support programs to treat anxiety, depression, and fatigue, as well as cognitive issues, (6) the Patient-2-Patient Network, a phone-based support program, in which a patient is paired with a fellow survivor of the same type of cancer to share their anxieties and concerns, (7) financial counseling, (8) Resource and Education Center (215-214-1618) providing educational seminars to the community on various health issues, and (9) social media, where patients post comments to connect with other patients online: Facebook, Twitter, Instagram.

Massachusetts General Hospital (MGH): Cancer Center Survivorship Program

55 Fruit Street, Boston, MA 02114
(617) 726-2000
massgeneral.org/cancer-center

The MGH Cancer Center Survivorship Program includes the following resources and services: (1) individual psychological services, (2) social workers who provide support regarding cancer-related issues affecting the patient and family members, as well as referrals to community resources, (3) the Network Peer Matching Program, a one-to-one support program where a patient is matched with another patient with a similar cancer diagnosis, treatment, and age, providing support due to shared experiences, often conducted over the phone, (4) the Oncology Sexual Health Clinic,

(5) the Katherine A. Gallagher Integrative Therapies Program which includes acupuncture, massage therapy, art and music therapy, qigong, and Tai Chi, (6) Lifestyle Medicine, which includes exercise, diet, stress management, and smoking cessation, designed to improve fitness, function, and quality of life, (7) one-to-one nutrition counseling, (8) mind-body skills resiliency groups (such as meditation and guided imagery), and (9) social media, where patients post comments to connect with other patients online: Facebook, Instagram, LinkedIn, YouTube.

MD Anderson Cancer Center

1515 Holcombe Boulevard, Houston, TX 77030
(877) 632-6789
mdanderson.org

MD Anderson Cancer Center offers the following services and resources: (1) survivorship clinics, (2) MyCancerConnection, which provides one-to-one support of patients who are matched with patients by disease site and type of treatment, conducted either in-person or over the telephone, (3) the Psychiatric Oncology Center, which provides support services to patients and family members, (4) PIKNIC, Partners in Knowledge News in a Cancer Survivorship Series, provides educational videos concerning cancer-related medical, psychological, and quality of life issues, (5) Integrative Medicine Center, which provides clinical services to reduce patients' distress and improve their emotional well-being (such as acupuncture, exercise classes, meditation), and (6) social media, where patients post comments to connect with other patients online: Facebook, Twitter, Pinterest, Instagram, LinkedIn, YouTube.

Memorial Sloan-Kettering Cancer Center: Adult Survivorship and Follow-Up Care Program

1275 York Avenue, New York, NY 10065
(800) 525-2225
mskcc.org

The Adult Survivorship and Follow-Up Care Program offers a broad range of services and resources for all cancer survivors: (1) disease-specific survivorship clinics for survivors of many cancer diagnoses, including those with the four cancer diagnoses included in this book (bladder, colorectal, non-Hodgkin lymphoma, and lung cancer), (2) identification and management of long-term and late side effects in the clinics, (3) individual and group counseling provided in-person and online, for both patients and caregivers, (4) a Patient-to-Patient support program, providing a linking of an individual patient to another patient with the same diagnosis, (5) lectures, seminars, and workshops which are conducted involving a wide range of topics, including information on both medical and nonmedical issues concerning the impact of cancer on survivors' lives (such as emotional, relationships with family and friends, financial), (6) MyMSK, an online program for family, caregivers and friends where they can get information about a patient's care, and (7) social media, where patients post comments online to connect with other patients: Facebook, Twitter, Pinterest, Instagram, LinkedIn, YouTube.

Moffitt Cancer Center: Survivorship Clinic

12902 USF Magnolia Drive, Tampa, FL 33612
(888) 663-3488
my.moffitt.org

Moffitt Cancer Center's Survivorship Clinic includes the following treatment, resources, and services: (1) a Survivorship Clinic, which includes (a) monitoring cancer spread, recurrence, and late effects, as well as prevention of recurrent and new cancers, (b) refocusing survivors on wellness issues, such as nutrition and exercise, (2) support groups for survivors and family members and friends, some of which are disease site-specific (such as lung, by telephone, and breast cancer, in-person, (3) social workers who meet individually with survivors, family members, and friends and recommend: (a) ways to manage stress, cope with the changes in their lives due to cancer, and (b) assist with transportation, lodging, and financial concerns, (4) online platforms for survivors and caregivers as a means to share their experiences with other survivors and caregivers, (5) Cardio-Oncology Program, which includes surveillance and treatment for those survivors with cardiotoxic side effects that may occur after treatment.

NYU Langone Hospital: Perlmutter Cancer Center Survivorship Program

160 East 34th Street, New York, NY 10016
(212) 731-6000
nyulangone.org

The Perlmutter Cancer Center Survivorship Program offers the following: (1) development of a care plan to optimize survivors' physical and emotional health after treatment and identifies resources for a healthy lifestyle, (2) social workers who provide help regarding family and financial issues, (3) referrals to a therapist to treat psychological problems, (4) one-on-one individual support and counseling by psychologists and social workers to help patients cope with having cancer, (5) educational programs that include lectures, panel discussions, and presentations by cancer specialists, health care professionals, survivors, and (6) CancerConnect, an online program for survivors and caregivers who write about the impact of cancer on their lives.

Stanford Cancer Survivorship Program

875 Blake Wilbur Drive, Palo Alto, CA 94304
(650) 498-6000
stanfordhealthcare.org/medical-clinical/cancer-survivorship-program.html

The Stanford Cancer Survivorship Program is designed to help survivors transition from diagnosis to wellness. It includes the following programs and resources: (1) personal consultations, (2) psychosocial care to treat post-cancer quality of life issues (such as psychological problems, family relationships), (3) support groups, (4) nutrition consults, (5) fitness classes, (6) workshops, (7) lectures, (8) the Stanford Center for Integrative Medicine, which offers complementary and alternative therapies, integrated with traditional medicine.

University of California at Los Angeles (UCLA): Jonsson Comprehensive Cancer Center

8-684 Factor Bldg., Box 951781, Los Angeles, CA 90095
(310) 825-5268
cancer.ucla.edu/patient-care/survivorship

The UCLA Jonsson Comprehensive Cancer Center includes the following services and resources for cancer survivors: (1) UCLA-LIVESTRONG VITA Program (Vital Information and Tailored Assessment), which develops survivorship care plans and identifies long-term and late cancer effects, (2) individual counseling of patients and family members by psychologists and social workers concerning psychological problems, (3) teaching mind-body techniques (e.g. relaxation and guided imagery), (4) the Looking Ahead Group, which connects survivors with other survivors who have completed treatment, (5) health promotion counseling, which is used to reduce the risk of health problems (such as weight gain, chronic diseases such as diabetes), (6) lectures and information on cancer-related topics held at the Cancer Center and provided online, and (7) internet links to outside survivorship resources.

University of California San Francisco (UCSF): Helen Diller Family Comprehensive Cancer Center

1450 3rd Street, San Francisco, CA 94158
(888) 689-8273
cancer.ucsf.edu

The UCSF Helen Diller Family Comprehensive Cancer Center offers a range of programs and services specific to cancer survivors as well as other services serving patients and survivors: (1) Survivorship Wellness Program, an eight-week clinical program involving psychologists, social workers, dieticians, and exercise counselors to help survivors optimize their wellness after finishing cancer treatment (such as psychological issues, physical activity, and nutrition, (tel: 415-353-3931), (2) support groups specific for survivors of the four cancers included in this book, as well as many others (tel: 415-353-9745), (3) individual consultation by a psychologist and psychiatrist concerning psychological issues and coping with having had cancer, (4) MyChart, used to reach patients' medical care team and medical information online, (5) peer support programs, in which patients are matched with volunteers similar to them in diagnosis, age, and gender, providing patients with comfort and support through shared experiences (tel: 415-885-3693), (6) the Cancer Resource Center, which provides information about cancer treatments, emotional support, and community resources (obtained online and in print), and (7) two eight-week workshops where patients share their personal experiences through art and writing.

REFERENCES

AHRQ (Agency for Healthcare Research and Quality). 2018. *2017 National Healthcare Quality and Disparities Report*. AHRQ Pub. No. 18-033-EF

Adorno G, Lopez E, Burg MA, Loerzel V, Killian M, Dailey AB, et al. 2018. Positive aspects of having had cancer: A mixed-methods analysis of responses from the American Cancer Society Study of Cancer Survivors-II (SCS-II). *Psycho-Oncology*, 27(5): 1412-1415

Beckjord EB, Arora NK, Bellizzi K, Hamilton AS, Rowland JH. 2011. Sexual well-being among survivors of non-Hodgkin lymphoma. *Oncology Nursing Forum*, 38(5): E351-E359

Burg MA, Adorno G, Lopez EDS, Loerzel V, Stein K, Wallace C, et al. 2015. Current unmet needs of cancer survivors: Analysis of open-ended responses to the American Cancer Society study of cancer survivors II. *Cancer* 121, 621–630

CancerCare. 2016. *CancerCare Patient Access and Engagement Report*, New York: CancerCare.

Chambers SK, Baade P, Youl P, Aitkin J, Occhipinti S, Vinod S, et al. 2015. Psychological distress and quality of life in lung cancer: The role of health-related stigma, illness appraisals and social constraints. *Psycho-Oncology* 24, 1569–1577

Dunn J, Ng SK, Breitbart W, Aitken J, Youl P, Baade PD, et al. 2013. Health-related quality of life and life satisfaction in colorectal cancer survivors: Trajectories of adjustment. *Health and Quality of Life Outcomes* 11, 46

Fiscella K, Sanders MR. 2016. Racial and ethnic disparities in the quality of health care. *Annual Review of Public Health* 37, 375–394

Green BL, Davis JL, Rivers D, Buchanan KL, Rivers B. 2014. Cancer health disparities. *In:* D. Alberts, LM Hess (eds) *Fundamentals of cancer prevention.* Springer-Verlag Berlin Heidelberg, 151–183

Jacobsen PB, Donovan KA, Trask PC, Fleishman SB, Zabora J, Baker F, Holland JC. 2005. Screening for psychological distress in ambulatory cancer patients. A multicenter evaluation of the Distress Thermometer. *Cancer* 103, 1494–1502

Jansen L, Hoffmeister M, Chang-Claude J, Brenner H, Arndt V. 2011. Benefit finding and post-traumatic growth in long-term colorectal cancer survivors: Prevalence, determinants, and associations with quality of life. *British Journal of Cancer* 105, 1158–1165

Kim Y, Carver CS, Spillers RL, Love-Ghaffari M, Kaw CK. 2012. Dyadic effects of fear of recurrence on the quality of life of cancer survivors and their caregivers. *Quality of Life Research* 21, 517–525

Kretschmer A, Grimm T, Buchner A, Stief CG, Karl A. 2016. Prognostic features for quality of life after radical cystectomy and orthotopic neobladder. *International Brazilian Journal of Urology* 42 (6): 1109–1120

Lowery AE, Krebs P, Coups EJ, Feinstein MB, Burkhalter JE, Park BJ, Ostroff JS. 2014. Impact of symptom burden in post-surgical non–small cell lung cancer survivors. *Supportive Care in Cancer* 22 (1): 173–180

National Cancer Institute, SEER Cancer Stat Facts https://seer.cancer.gov/data/citation.html

Parikh-Patel A, Morris CR, Kizer KW. 2017. Disparities in quality of cancer care: The role of health insurance and population demographics. *Medicine* 96: 50, e9125

Reeve BB, Potosky AL, Smith AW, Han PK, Hays RD, Davis WW, et al. 2009. Impact of cancer on health-related quality of life of older Americans. *Journal of the National Cancer Institute* 101, 860–868

Sarker S-J, Smith SK, Chowdhury K, Ganz PA, Zimmerman S, Gribben J, Korszun A. 2017. Comparison of the impact of cancer between the British and US long-term non-Hodgkin lymphoma survivors. *Supportive Care in Cancer* 25 (3): 739–748

Smith SK, Mayer DK, Zimmerman S, Williams CS, Benecha H, Ganz PA, et al. 2013. Quality of life among long-term survivors of non-Hodgkin lymphoma: A follow-up study. *Journal of Clinical Oncology* 31 (2): 272–279

INDEX

For the benefit of digital users, indexed terms that span two pages (e.g., 52–53) may, on occasion, appear on only one of those pages.